MORE ADVANCE PRAISE FOR CANCER ETIQUETTE

Cancer Etiquette is a helpful layman's guide as to how the author feels you can beneficially act, if you or a close friend or loved one has cancer. It suggests ways to think about and discuss the illness and associated problems, as well as support the patient in confronting what is often a devastating event in their life. It emphasizes the support structure available, that many people share similar problems, and that they are not alone. It is a forthright way of thinking about the many difficulties that arise and how the author suggests these can be handled.

Murry G. Fischer, M.D., F.A.C.S.

If you have ever struggled with what to say to a friend or relative diagnosed with cancer, I highly recommend Rosanne Kalick's book, *Cancer Etiquette*. Using insights gleaned from personal experience as a cancer survivor, interviews with cancer patients, and extensive research, the author steers us through the difficulties of knowing or living with the people who have been diagnosed or treated for cancer. It is written with clarity, humor, and sensitivity.

Joan Milano, MSW, psychoanalyst

My years of experience have taught me that there is no one "right" way to communicate. Each person is different and has needs that are unique.

During one of her treatment sessions Rosanne told me she had a follow-up and was waiting for results. I replied, "Oh, don't worry; it will be fine," my usual trite comeback, when patients were awaiting test results. Her reply was, "Are you sure?" This one simple comment has changed the way I talk to patients waiting for test results. I, like they, can't be sure. I can hope, I can pray, and I can ask if and why they are worried, but I can't shut down the communication with canned answers.

This book is one that every person who has been touched by cancer, whether personally or professionally, should read.

Kathleen Duffy, Administrative Director
Cancer Program-Dickstein Cancer Center,
White Plains Hospital, White Plains, New York

CANCER
Etiquette

CANCER
Etiquette

What to Say
A Neighbor

What to Do
A Colleague

When Someone You Know
A Stranger   A Friend

or Love Has Cancer
A Relative   A Loved One

ROSANNE KALICK

This is a Lion Book.

Lion Books and its logo are trademarks of Lion Books Publisher.

Lion Books Publisher titles may be purchased for business or promotional use or for special sales. Discounts on book quantities are available. For information, please contact Lion Books Publisher.

PRINTED IN THE UNITED STATES OF AMERICA

This book was edited by Harriet Ross.

Book design by Lisa Sloane

Jacket design by Susan Zucker

Library of Congress Control Number: 2004112012

ISBN 0-87460-450-8

10   9   8   7   6   5   4   3   2   1

First edition published 2005.

Names used in stories have been changed to protect privacy.

A portion of the proceeds of this book will be donated to cancer research and education.

For

Alex, Maddie, Sydney, Henry and Josh.

Grandma will love you forever and ever.

CONTENTS

FIRST WORDS

How do we protect and enhance the dignity of our friend who has cancer? How do we promote the emotional connection so crucial to living and recovering or, indeed, even to dying well? Common sense goals, but very uncomfortable territory for most of us. Packed into Rosanne Kalick's book are words and suggestions that help—they leap from her every page. Many are common sense; all come from the insights of an acutely aware woman who has been there.

This author has it right. We "outsiders" WANT intensely to help. We want NOT to hurt, NOT to be frozen by our own fears. Talking and doing for the cancer patient are not automatic for most of us. Ms. Kalick pulls down the barriers and lets us see the many ways, often very simple ways, that will make the difference.

Ms. Kalick emphasizes the crucial step for the cancer patient of returning to one's life plan where one's cancer plan does not dominate. Her insights point the way for us to help and to identify obstacles. The patients, who are our relatives and friends, will bless her, first for telling their story, and then, even more so, when we listen and learn from it.

Rosanne has lived the cancer life. She knows first hand the pain and the fear, what hurts, and what retards progress. She also knows what works. With that insight, she leads the rest of us to see, to understand, and, above all, to be able to help. Thank you, Rosanne.

Maurice J. Mahoney, MD, JD
Professor of Genetics, Pediatrics, and Obstetrics & Gynecology
Yale University School of Medicine

1

MY PERSONAL DOUBLE WHAMMY (OR HOW I CAME TO WRITE THIS BOOK)*

"You have cancer."

Hearing those words once is bad. Twice is devastating.

This is not a "how-to" book. Having lived through two agonizing battles with two different cancers, I am expert only in the struggle for my own survival. But I also lived through the comments, queries, reactions, and behavior of strangers, friends, and family toward me as the comfortable world I thought I knew was totally transformed. Having cancer changes people. This book grew out of those changes and their influences on me: the rude or cruel appraisals of my physical appearance, the sometimes stupid attempts to be humorous, the well-meaning but thoughtless stabs at being helpful. A phrase leapt out at me—*Cancer Etiquette*—and I immediately knew that should be the book's title.

Now, mind you, in all fairness, many people uttered comforting, soothing words; many people knew just what to do when I was desperate and confused. My family was as solidly supportive as they could be; but there were enough blunders and enough hurtful mishaps to make me wonder if perhaps other cancer patients had felt verbally abused, or had endured behavioral "boo-boos." So, I started asking. And did they ever come forth with their resentments, their pain, and their anger!

Although some had positive memories, too many others recounted incidents that caused anguish and deep hurt. Then I knew I was onto something. I pursued my research with voluminous reading of books and articles on cancer and its impact on people. I also communicated through e-mails and interviews with patients and caregivers from all over the

---

*At the end of this book, in the *Afterword* section, I have recounted the story of my cancers.

country and, in some cases, outside the United States. All the stories in this book are true, even though some incidents sound almost unbelievable. Full names, of course, are not given for reasons of privacy.

The more I investigated, the more convinced I became that most people do not know what to say or what to do when someone they know or love has cancer. This book will help them to find words that will not offend or hurt, but will help to comfort. This book will enable them to perform simple acts of loving-kindness that are blessings to the patient.

If you become more aware of the power your words have to hurt—or heal, this book will have accomplished its purpose. If you become more knowing about how to help—not hinder—the recovery of someone who is battling cancer, then we can all say, "Hooray!"

2 YESTERDAY'S LANGUAGE

Say "Dread disease," and everyone knows what you're talking about. Say "The Big C," and no one doubts that the phrase is shorthand for cancer. The word, cancer, used to be so taboo that people feared saying it. Cancer has always been thought of as something insidious that eats away at us. As early as 1651, cancer not only was a malignancy; it represented evil. It is no wonder, therefore, that the word *cancer* has such power, evokes such fear, that the capital "C" is enough to communicate.

The illness has a long history. Ancient Egyptian medical papyri dating to 3000 B.C. describe tumors. Mummified Inca remains from 2400 years ago suggest the presence of the skin cancer melanoma. There is evidence of breast cancer in a specimen dating from the Bronze Age. Herodotus and Hippocrates mention cancer in their writings. There is even a patron of cancer patients, St. Peregrine, who lived in the 14th century.

Cancer affects us as does no other disease. Years ago, if cancer was mentioned at all, it was done in a whisper. In truth, not so long ago, a diagnosis of cancer often was a death sentence. Ellen Leopold in her history of breast cancer, *A Darker Ribbon*, speaks of how cancer patients were scapegoated. "As both carriers and victims of malevolent spirit, they had to be cast out, as a spell."

You have cancer. You represent my worst fears. You make me think of my own mortality. You make me think of my mother, or father, or friend who had cancer and died. Cancer, the disease of out-of-control cells, is what we fear the most. Will my body, too, go out of control?

In the 1950s, two women, Teresa Lasser and Fanny Rosenow, who later founded Reach to Recovery, had mastectomies. They wanted to place an ad in *The New York Times* announcing a forum where women could speak about breast cancer. They were told that the *Times* would not publish the word "breast" or "cancer" in the notice. Today, speaking or writing about cancer is encouraged. Today, we can consider early detection a potential life sentence, not a death sentence.

Patients, therapists, medical personnel, and clergy are writing about cancer. Go into any bookstore and you will find a large selection of books dealing with every aspect of the disease. There are survivor stories, books on particular cancers, traditional treatment options, nutrition, and alternative medicine.

TODAY'S LANGUAGE

Many writers have used metaphor in an attempt to communicate the power cancer has on all of us. Novelist Alice Hoffman wrote that upon hearing of her cancer diagnosis, "In a single moment, the world as I knew it dropped away from me, leaving me on a far and distant planet, one where there was no gravity and no oxygen and nothing made sense anymore."

Alice Trillin, a non-smoker, had lung cancer when she was thirty-eight years old. Surgeons removed a lobe; radiation and chemotherapy followed. Fourteen years later, a persistent cough caused Trillin to worry. Had the lung cancer returned? She writes in *The New Yorker* of cancer as a dragon. ". . . we can never kill this dragon, but we go about the business of our daily lives—giving our children breakfast, putting more mulch on our gardens—in the hope that it will stay asleep for a while longer."

Cancer requires strong language, and a common metaphor is that of a battleground. This image calls up the ferocity of dealing with the disease. Battles can go on for days, weeks, months, or years. The same is true of cancer. In war, there is fear, pain, loss, confusion, anger, and occasional retreat. There are command centers. In the operating room, the surgeon works in the "field." A bone marrow transplant is a rescue. In battle, some lose and some win. Surviving one skirmish does not mean the battle is won.

Since September 11, 2001, terrorism has become all too real. We are all much more careful as we look around us. We accept delays and searches at airports. Although terrorism does not control our lives, it certainly is present on our emotional radar screen. Cancer is like a terrorist attack. There is usually no warning. We don't know where it will strike. Cancer symptoms, if there are any, often start innocuously. Those of us who survive the cancer attack nevertheless are permanently affected by it. The cancer terrorist lurks even when we are in remission. Will another attack occur? How can I protect myself? What should I do in case of another attack? I have to accept the fear; I must acknowledge its presence. In terms of September 11, I try to live my life as though the terrorists will not attack. If I cower, if I fail to engage in life, if fear becomes paramount, the terrorist wins.

I have my own personal metaphors. One, in particular, is that of a Marathon. Before my diagnosis, I had completed three New York City marathons. I knew that my cancer treatment would take a year and a half to complete. I couldn't grasp that concept, so I used the 26-mile run as my metaphor. Each series of treatments became one leg of the marathon. VAD, a standard chemotherapy cocktail, was the segment from Staten Island over the Verazanno Bridge. Another chemical cocktail consisting of four drugs, EDAP, was the trek across Brooklyn. The harvesting of the stem cells occurred as I crossed the Pulaski Bridge. At about 20 miles in any marathon, the runner usually "hits the wall." It is the moment when the body rebels; there is nothing left—no energy, no muscle capable of working, nothing but pain. The body rebels at what it's been forced to endure; yet the runner continues. That is what the transplant process is like. By the time I completed the second stem cell transplant, I had crossed the cancer marathon finish line, exhausted, yet knowing I had achieved victory.

Today, since we speak more freely about cancer, it is time to acknowledge that the words we use, and the things we do, play important roles in patient recovery. The cliché about "sticks and stones" is simply not true; words can and do harm us. I learned this the hard way. Since cancer has become more a chronic and less a fatal disease, it's time that we acknowledge the effect that hearing about a cancer diagnosis, whether it's our own or that of someone we know, has on our ability to speak and to act. It's time to acknowledge that our words can heal or hurt, and that our fear impedes our ability to communicate about cancer. Let's take cancer out of the proverbial darkness!

Sooner or later, if it hasn't already happened, someone you know, someone you love, or someone in your workplace will say, "I have cancer." How will you respond? What will you say? What will you do?

Everyone wants to say and do the right thing. Not everyone succeeds. The effect of cancer on the patient is obvious. The effect on friends, coworkers, and family is less evident, but, nevertheless, very important.

WORDS THAT HURT

When I was first diagnosed with multiple myeloma, I was the Chairperson of the Library and Learning Resource Center at Westchester Community College in Valhalla, New York. I decided to inform the other librarians and staff before my condition became public knowledge on campus. It was difficult to tell them I had cancer, to explain what this strange cancer was, and that the treatment would be lengthy. Their reactions were powerful. We were family.

One librarian came up to me afterward, and quietly told me how wonderful hospice was. I hadn't even started treatment. That was my first experience with words that hurt. I know that librarian cared about me. I know she meant well. Her mother had recently died in hospice, and I assume that's what provoked her reaction. She was remembering death; I was just beginning to cope with the reality of the medical challenges to come.

A few days later, another member of the college family came into my office. Her casual comment was, "Don't you know you're ruining everyone's Thanksgiving?" I may have said, "I don't give a shit." If I didn't, I wish I had. This colleague also meant no harm, but her words failed. She spoke without thinking of the power her words might have on me. Perhaps this was her poor attempt at humor; I didn't hear it that way. Perhaps it was her inept effort to tell me that many people cared about me. Whatever her motivation, she failed to convey that. I realize now, as I did not then, that cancer can have this effect on one's ability to communicate. I do not know why cancer has this power. It's almost as though the disease strikes our verbal immune system. Too often in life we speak without thinking. However, careless words about cancer cannot be recalled as we recall faulty tires.

Years after my treatment for multiple myeloma, I was diagnosed with breast cancer. I called one friend, someone I've known for more than 40 years. She's extremely bright, and very funny. I told her I needed a double mastectomy. Her immediate response was, "At least you'll be symmetrical." I told her that I could say something like that, but she couldn't. She knew immediately she had spoken inappropriately. Perhaps, caught in her emotional reaction to the situation, she was trying to push away the news with black humor. Still, it was hurtful.

That evening, I called another friend. She became hysterical on the phone. "YOU'VE GOT WHAT? I DON'T BELIEVE IT." She, too, meant no harm. The diagnosis was just too much for her. I had to calm her down. Both of these friends had traveled to Little Rock to keep me company years earlier as I underwent the multiple myeloma treatment—they were not casual acquaintances. Overwhelmed emotionally, friends, family, colleagues, even significant others may not be able to focus on the person with cancer. Instead, they are dealing with their own visceral reactions.

THE POWER OF WORDS

There are more than 1,300,000 cases of cancer diagnosed in the United States annually. That's one new case every 25 seconds. Think of the words involved, diagnoses made, consultations needed, treatment plans to consider. And those are only the medical words. Think of the words of anger, frustration, fear, and pain, of the words needed to communicate to friends and family, to colleagues, even to insurance companies. Think of the unsaid, words too frightening to speak.

Behind every cancer diagnosis is a story. Every case is different, every person unique, every family constellation special. There are those who are totally alone. Others are surrounded by support. Therefore, there can be no hard and fast rules. What I have learned, though, is that people do want guidance. "I don't know what to say; I don't know what to do," are all-too-common pleas for help.

3
WHAT WE SAY AND HOW WE SAY IT

Words can build us up; words can tear us down. Cancer tears the patient down physically; the power of the words of friends and loved ones can strengthen. Surgery, although traumatic, heals. Radiation and chemotherapy make the patient very ill, but those processes also heal. During treatment, when the immune system is compromised, the emotional immune system is also weakened. We need to be careful of how we speak lest we unintentionally do harm to the person we want most to help.

If you're going for a job interview, you're likely to imagine questions that might be asked, and plan your answers. You may take written notes to a department meeting, if there is an agenda item you expect to comment on. At any committee meeting, you'll probably consider your response before you raise your hand to speak. Even if you return a garment to a department store, you'll have some sort of explanation in mind as you meet with the salesperson. Yet, when it comes to hearing of a cancer diagnosis, a damaging verbal artery often opens. Joseph Telushkin, writing in *Words That Hurt: Words That Heal*, says, "The time to avoid making ugly comments is before they leave your mouth. Once they do, the other party might forgive; it is unlikely that he or she will forget."

CAN YOU BELIEVE ANYONE WOULD SAY THAT?

At a luncheon, during a lull in conversation, one guest hears another saying, "Don't drink from Sally's cup; she has cancer." Aside from being scientific hogwash, since cancer is certainly not contagious, this comment only perpetuates a medical myth.

On another occasion, a newly diagnosed patient hears her friend say, "I know how you must be feeling. My sisters had cancer. Neither of them made it." And, unbelievably, a woman whose daughter was diagnosed with breast cancer sent her a sympathy card and wrote in it, "Goodbye." What purpose is served with remarks like these except to heighten the patient's anxiety? Intentional or not, the words are damaging.

Miriam K. was in the hospital recovering from surgery for ovarian cancer. The phone rang; it was her mother-in-law. She asked Miriam if the hospital would provide hospice care for "later," or if they would just "drop" her. Those weren't the words Miriam needed to hear at that time. Knowing her mother-in-law, she wasn't that surprised at the comments, but we can be shocked. Miriam had had major surgery; she was facing months of chemotherapy; she was worried about her husband and two teenage daughters. She was certainly not thinking of hospice. End-of-life issues are certainly not the issues to be addressed within hours of a patient's major surgery or within a few days of diagnosis or treatment. Never deny hope.

Beth Murphy, in *Fighting for Our Future*, writes about a young woman who, after telling a friend she had breast cancer, got the following response, "Oh, my, what's your husband going to do without you?" First, it appears as though this individual assumed the patient was going to die. The truth is that today, cancer is more likely to be a chronic rather than a fatal disease. Second, the friend should have focused her attention on the patient at that moment, not on the husband.

In another instance, a 12-year-old boy in treatment for leukemia had his photo taken with Andre Agassi. His mother proudly shared the photo with a group of friends. All were positive about the snapshot, commenting on how lucky the boy and his mom were to meet Agassi, and how handsome Agassi was. However, one person looking at the snapshot said, "It almost makes it worth getting leukemia, doesn't it!" Really?

Another hard-to-believe account: James G. is a lawyer. Because of all the tests he had to undergo, he was unable to call a client for four days. The client was furious. James explained that he had been unable to get to the office, that he had just been diagnosed with cancer. The furious client said, "Good—you got what you deserve."

Mike S. runs a large auto maintenance and repair facility. A customer he had served for eight years came in and said, "I hear that you have cancer so I am going to start looking for a new mechanic now." Mike tore up the customer's work order and told him to start looking. Good for Mike.

Another patient, Greg R., heard words that hurt him. He said his employer treated him like "dirt" and his sister had "zip empathy" for him.

Though he had extensive treatment, he did not go into remission. To compound matters, Greg's sister was angry because it was she who had to assume the major responsibility for their elderly mother. In an outraged tone, she said to him, "How dare you use cancer as an excuse?" His greatest support came from strangers he met on an Internet cancer list. In this case, his family totally failed him.

So can a friend's words fail. Annette was recovering from a transplant and was still extremely tired. Nevertheless, she was trying to work part time. A friend, a smoker, offered her a ride to work. When Annette asked her to open the car window so that the smoke would dissipate, her friend's response was, "Why? You already have cancer."

Linda M.'s former classmate made an equally insensitive remark. Hearing that Linda had been diagnosed with cancer, he called and said, "I hear you're leaving us." Linda was silent for a few moments and then responded, "Where am I going?"

What is the patient to think? Does the classmate think Linda is going to die? Is he merely trying to be funny? Does he know something Linda doesn't? In this instance, Linda chose to answer literally. What made this conversation particularly disturbing was that Linda had not heard from this high school friend for 35 years. How could he have made such a remark? Remember: what you may think of as an idle comment may be interpreted more seriously than you intended.

Similarly, a casual acquaintance asked someone who had recently had a colostomy, "Are the bags you use paper or plastic?" Intrusive and embarrassing. I might have responded, "None of your damned business." A more controlled response might be, "That's too personal to ask." There are some questions a casual acquaintance does not have the right to ask.

Family members, too, must be sensitive with the words they use. A "woman of a certain age," a friend of a friend, needed a mastectomy. A distant but loving cousin, in an attempt to be supportive, said to her, "So what if you lose it? It's only an appendage. You don't need it anymore, do you? You can live without it." He continued to play down the importance of "it" so that the loss of her breast wouldn't matter. However, she had to make up her own mind that she had absolutely no choice. She was numb but accepting, and resigned to surgery.

This incident offers food for thought. First, would a woman have spoken the way the man did, even as a loving cousin? Breasts represent so much to a woman: her sexuality, her femininity, nourishment for her children. A woman's response might have been markedly different. She might have said to him, "A breast is not merely an appendage. It's a major part of my body, of my life. I know I have to have the mastectomy, but I expect more understanding about how big a loss this will be for me." Second, the cousin could have been more careful with his words, saying something like, "You're my cousin. I'll love you even if you have only one breast. I want you to live, and if that means you have to have a mastectomy, then please do it."

Then, too, the patient has some responsibility in the decision making (as when she realized she had no choice regarding the surgery). Admittedly, everyone faces cancer differently. The gamut runs from those who totally immerse themselves in cancer research to those who deal only with minimal details, the "whatever-the-doctor says-I'll-do" approach. It is much too subjective an issue to generalize about. Ours is not to judge which is the better approach. The issue is which of the two options offers the most comfort to the patient.

Less intrusive, but equally upsetting, are close friends who make verbal gaffes. Terry's words failed when Linda E. most needed her support. Linda had undergone five chemotherapy treatments. Her cancer markers, blood tests the physician uses to track to see if the patient is responding to treatment, were improving. In spite of the common side effects—nausea, baldness, loss of her eyebrows and eyelashes—she was optimistic. What Linda wanted at this time was to hear some supporting words from her friend. She would have preferred silence to Terry's comment, "Oh, chemo is cumulative! You'll feel much worse later on." Granted, Terry may have been right, but what purpose did those words serve? We need to filter our words so we don't inadvertently destroy optimism.

Sometimes when we speak, we miscommunicate. Patients preparing for surgery, undergoing treatment or waiting for test results are often tense and hypersensitive. For example, Nicole has a brain tumor. She is divorced and has one daughter. The night before surgery, she saw her ex-husband who said, "Does this mean I get Maria when you die?" The fact that he made the comment with a straight face indicated to Nicole that he was serious. Perhaps he was trying to lighten Nicole's mood. If he was, he failed. She was very upset and responded, "No, because I'm going to outlive you." If he was serious, the evening before surgery was hardly the right time to bring up the issue of their child's future.

You would expect sensitivity from medical personnel, but this is not necessarily the case. Natalie Davis Singarn tells of one medical resident who made an effort to communicate with a young woman awaiting discharge after a mastectomy. He noted the books on her night table, observed that she must enjoy reading, and said, "Well, you should read *On Death and Dying.*"

MORE STORIES

Barbara Gamarekian had peritoneal cancer, a form of abdominal cancer. She, too, knew that sometimes people say the strangest things. Barbara wrote of her experience at a wedding brunch. A woman she knew approached, pointed her finger skyward and said, "Harry is waiting for you up there!" Harry, her husband, had been dead for about a year. Such a comment would have seemed ludicrous on a sitcom. Barbara managed to respond. "I hope Harry has a long wait."

Gamarekian belonged to a summer tennis club, a club with a long waiting list. The membership fee was $1,000, and Gamarekian played doubles every week. The manager was an old friend and sympathetic when she called to explain her situation, and why she had not responded to the renewal mailing. Still, after a pause, he asked, "So what do you plan to do about your tennis membership?" His was a legitimate question, but it was absolutely the wrong time to persist with it.

What prompts such remarks? Probably the words come out because the individuals really don't know what to say. Barbara has cancer. Cancer can kill. Harry is dead. Therefore, if B follows A, then on some level the observer saw a connection. If Barbara has a Stage III cancer, maybe she will give up her tennis membership. There's a long waiting list for membership, so why not ask?

Eleanor was suffering from advanced pancreatic cancer. A renewal application from her country club arrived in the mail. When she approached her husband about the decision, he said, "What's the point of rejoining? You're not going to live long enough to enjoy it." Literally, her husband's words were accurate. Granted, country club membership can be expensive, but his words certainly fell far short of the kind and supportive response she needed. He should have said something like, "Sure, let's take a chance; get in as much golf as you can." He might even have said, "I'll call the club; maybe we can sign up for six months and then extend the membership. I want you to spend as much time as possible on the course." A third response could have been, "I hope you'll be well enough to play at the club, but do you think, given the medical situation, we should rejoin?" Did he intend to raise the red flag to his wife, indicating how little time she had left? Maybe, maybe not. Had he paused for just a few seconds, he might have succeeded rather than failed with his words. Eleanor spent many of her last half-well days alone, at a public course, playing her favorite game of golf.

These examples, admittedly, are extremes. People do say outrageous things. Most lapses are less obvious; nevertheless, we must try to avoid them. When I was diagnosed with breast cancer, someone I knew only slightly said, "If anyone should have this, it's you." She quickly realized what she had said and apologized. What had been meant as a compliment came across miserably. I had already dealt with one cancer, so it seemed natural to her that I would handle this second cancer as well. Even if that were true, what could she gain by saying those words? She simply needed to fill a verbal vacuum, and that can be dangerous.

Even a look can communicate negatively. Many women report that after telling someone about their breast cancer, they instantly notice the visual breast check that some people make. Which breast was removed? Which breast was treated?

Kathy B.'s husband, Chuck, had multiple myeloma. Her friend called to tell her how wonderful Geraldine Ferraro looked when she appeared on the *Today* show, shortly after she had announced she was under treatment for the disease. Kathy did not need to hear her friend say, "She looks fantastic! She says she feels great. How come Chuck looks so bad?" Those remarks accomplish nothing, and cause anguish to the patient.

The fact that someone was once a cancer patient doesn't guarantee immunity from verbal blunders. A young breast cancer patient got a call from a neighbor in town who also had been treated for the disease. Instead of offering encouragement or help, the neighbor told her how glad she was to find out that another woman had a prognosis worse than hers.

One would think that those who routinely deal with cancer patients would be particularly sensitive to their needs. Surprisingly, even they can still be thoughtless. A friend was in a shop that sells bathing suits, lingerie, and breast prostheses. As she was looking through the bathing suit section, a young woman entered, and one saleswoman said in a loud voice to a saleswoman across the floor, "This is a new mastectomy customer." Turning to the woman, she said, "You are new, aren't you?" First, the comment should not have been so loud that another person could overhear it. It's difficult enough to go for a prosthesis fitting. This is a particularly private experience. I asked the fitter at the shop where I go what she would have done. She suggests that the salespeople speak quietly. Second, if another customer is nearby, she says, "I have a special customer here," or "Please take this woman to our specialty area." In the earlier instance, why couldn't the salesperson simply walk the young woman to the fitting area? Her privacy would then have been preserved.

Privacy is important. Brian L. and his wife went to a university library to get a book on caregiving for their son, whose 32-year-old wife had recently been diagnosed with breast cancer. The librarian shouted to an assistant on the other side of the room, "They need a book on care for cancer victims." Brian instantly protested, claiming his daughter-in-law wasn't a "victim." Brian was right; cancer patients aren't victims. The librarian and the saleswoman need to remember that they are professionals, and they must act professionally. They need to be reminded that some issues are confidential, that it is common courtesy not to speak aloud about confidential issues, that the needs of the customer, however that is defined, always come first.

Rita K.'s experience reminds us not only of the importance of our words, but also of our tone of voice. She was nearing the checkout line when a distant relative who was in line shouted, "You look so GOOD!" Her voice was loud enough so that others turned to look. Leaning toward her, but in a voice still loud enough for others to hear, the relative asked, "Are you in remission?" Rita noted that all the relative had to say was, "Hi, so good to see you." Rita would then have told her what was going on in her life and volunteer the information she wanted to give. The relative was rude in shouting across the aisle; she was rude in her comment; she was rude in her question about remission. Public places are public places. Private conversations should take place in private, or, if *both* parties are willing to talk in public, they should speak quietly. The conversation should be for two, not for all.

No one intentionally wants to hurt another, especially under circumstances where cancer is involved. It may be that you realize you could be in this situation instead of me. It may be that you don't want your friend, loved one, or colleague to die, but you just can't say that. It may just be the shock of the news. Whatever the cause, if we know that the period immediately following diagnosis is likely to cause us to misspeak, then we can prepare ourselves accordingly. Think before you speak, lest you come out with a meaningless—or worse, hurtful—cliché. If you feel the need to express yourself, just say, "I'm sorry."

Lila Keary has a spectacular sense of humor and a perfect ear for the cancer clichés we hear so often. Among the phrases she can do without are: "Things could be worse," "If it's meant to be, it's meant to be," and the phrase she hates most, "Years from now we'll look back at this and laugh." She suggests that if you can't talk, listen and "be in charge of Kleenex distribution."

Probably a separate book could be written on the lack of consideration by some insurance company representatives. I was in the hospital in Little Rock, the evening before a scheduled stem cell transplant. My insurance company had paid for the chemotherapy, as well as for the stem cell removal. Yet, that night I got a call from the hospital's finance office telling me that the insurance company was refusing to pay for the transplant itself. That was great news with which to embark on a life-threatening procedure.

In another instance, an insurance company representative told the patient she should have a fund-raiser because they weren't going to pay for her transplant. In the case of insurance companies, simple words can literally kill—for example, "Treatment denied."

Helen V.'s experience differed from mine; her insurance carrier did better. The stereotype is of the insurer questioning every claim, every test, any request for a consultation. Helen's case manager was kind and compassionate. When Helen called, the manager tried to expedite the resolution of her questions. When this particular manager left for a position elsewhere, she called Helen to tell her how good her replacement was, and that she shouldn't worry. The insurance company reduced stress, instead of causing it. It can happen.

LOOKING GOOD

Even a simple phrase may not be simple. Many times during my treatment I was told, "You look great." Compared to what? My friends weren't going to tell me I looked awful. One cancer patient, in Elise Babcock's book, *When Life Becomes Precious*, said, "I know I don't look great—I can see it in the mirror. But I'm doing the best I can. I'm wearing this wig to spare their feelings, to make it easier on them, because they can't deal with my bald head or the cancer. What I really want them to say is, 'I know you feel like hell. Please feel free to talk about it with me.' " A comment for a man might be, "I notice that you shaved today;" to a woman, "I like the lipstick you're wearing."

When Carole L. was told, "You look so good," she wondered, "How am I supposed to look?" The "You look so good" line seems to be used more with cancer patients than with those who have other medical problems. After major surgery of any kind, patients do not "look good," and no one is likely to say they do. Why do people feel the need to make such a comment to a cancer patient? The comment usually comes when someone meets a person who is undergoing chemotherapy. Many cancer patients look pale during treatment. Others lose weight. There are those who look tired, others who look pained, literally and figuratively. The faces of many may be swollen if they are receiving steroids as part of the protocol. For the most part, the cancer patient receiving chemotherapy does not look good.

Lois, whose experiences are discussed in Chapter 11 of this book, recalls that at several family get-togethers, her mother-in-law, of whom Lois is very fond, would genuinely express her concern and ask, "How are you feeling?" Lois's response was an often abrupt, but truthful, "lousy" or similar negative expression. Mom's response, "But you look so good." Lois hated that comment more than any other. How she looked was the result of a lot of effort. Although she appreciated the sentiment, she really resented the platitude.

Perhaps such comments are made because the speaker really didn't know what to expect. True, some patients are bedridden during part of each treatment cycle. Consequently, if an individual sees that the patient is alert and functioning, the instinct may be to say, "You look great." Resist the urge. Don't romanticize how the patient looks.

I'd like to suggest some options. The patient may have worked very hard to look as good as possible knowing, as Lois did, that inside she felt lousy. Consider saying, "I'm glad to see that you're doing so well in spite of the chemo." If it's not the first time you've seen the patient, you could say, "You look so much better than you did a week ago." Even "You're looking stronger—how are you dealing with the treatment?" can work. When the patient finishes treatment and seems to be regaining strength, then you can honestly say, "You look terrific." Say it when it's true, not when you want it to be true.

I suggest that we imagine ourselves talking into a tape recorder. On playback, would those be the words we'd really want to say? If you remember the image of the tape recorder, then think carefully before you permit yourself to hit the record button. What would you want said to you if the cancer role were reversed?

AVOIDING ERRORS

We've all made verbal mistakes. The goal is to lessen our chances for verbal blunders. The most likely time for error occurs when a family member, friend, or colleague tells of his diagnosis. Casual acquaintances usually find out after the dust has settled, but those closest to the situation, whether prepared or not, are likely to react viscerally. Even the period before the test results come in may be a volatile one. If, for example, you say to your friend who's awaiting biopsy results, "It's nothing," you're denying the very real anxiety felt by the person awaiting those results.

As one who was told by many, "It's nothing," and found out twice that "nothing" was really *something*, I recommend saying, "It's likely to be nothing serious," or "I hope it's nothing." This changes wishful thinking into a reality check. It may not be wise to say, "You'll be fine." "You'll probably be fine" is a better choice. The first statement makes you sound omnipotent. Of course, you want the patient to be fine. You can't deal with the possibility that she won't be fine any more than she can. Assuming everything will be all right, however, doesn't give the patient "wiggle room." How can he speak to you of his fears of treatment, of dying, of disfigurement, if you say everything will be fine? It shuts down the communication artery, which is exactly what you don't want to do. Changing one word can change the tone of the message.

Remember that waiting for test results gives new meaning to Einstein's theory of relativity. This is a particularly stressful time. The cancer clock is on for the patient.

There are no absolutes, just guidelines. One size does not fit all. One guideline may be that less is more. Pause before you speak. It's perfectly OK to say, "I don't know what to say." There is no single perfect response, no litany for proper speech. Everyone is in a state of shock when a diagnosis is made. The patient, too, may not know what to say. Your response could be as simple as "I'm sorry to hear that." If you're a close friend or member of the family, an expletive may communicate what you need to say. A hug may be just the right response.

A screaming toddler is told by his parents, "Use your words." We need to do the same. Although cancer is no longer the silent disease, it still, in many instances, strangles us verbally and emotionally. It should not be a disease of miscommunication as well as runaway cells.

HOW ARE YOU?

I would be remiss if I did not include a reference here to the question most commonly asked of the patient, "How are you?" There is inherently nothing wrong with such a question. But is it the standard "How are you?" we routinely ask when we aren't really interested in the answer? Is it the mundane "How are you?" where the expected reply is the one word "fine," or "OK?" Or is the actual question, "How are you, really?" A variation could be "How are you today?" This permits focus on a cancer snapshot rather than the entire album. Recovery is measured in small steps. Just adding the word *today* may give your friend an opportunity to indicate progress in the last 24 hours. Conversely, if it's been a bad day, you both are speaking of only one day; the implication is that tomorrow might be a better day. In any case, if you ask the question, be prepared for the real answer. The question does connote caring and concern. It is often the way that communication starts. In general, if you're not prepared for the answer, don't ask the question.

It's critical that even the "How are you?" question be an open-ended one. As a patient, I needed to know there would be space for my truth, my words, whether they were upbeat or not. The "How are you?" question should give me the opportunity to speak of my fear, concerns, and even anger. We may all be in denial about cancer at times, but as a friend, caregiver, loved one, you need to let me know that I can have my moments of truth, painful as those moments might be. Good words can do that.

CAN YOU BE TOO POSITIVE?

Another statement cancer patients often hear is "You have to be positive." How could that be a bad thing to say? In *The Human Side of Cancer*, a patient speaking to Dr. Jimmie Holland commented, "If any more people tell me to think positive, I'm going to slug them." Why should a person who has cancer have to think positively all the time? Even in our non-cancer lives there are times when we feel depressed, frustrated, or annoyed. When a child falls and scrapes his knee, he isn't told to be positive. You take care of the scrape at the same time you're comforting the child. The wound takes time to heal. Why should we do less with someone wounded by cancer? Doesn't overemphasizing the importance of a positive attitude imply that a negative attitude makes the disease worse? The reality is that some with negative attitudes survive while others with a positive attitude don't. We need to have reasonable expectations for the patient. Don't expect someone with cancer, recovering from surgery, chemotherapy, or radiation, to be strong all the time.

That's a big demand for anyone. Dr. Holland calls this the "tyranny of positive thinking." There's nothing wrong with positive thinking, of course, if it works for that particular patient at that particular moment. Are you positive all the time? Perhaps people want the patient to be positive because it makes them feel more comfortable. This positive thinking overkill can be typified in the remark, "You are lucky it is not worse." One breast cancer patient said, "Frankly, being thirty-six and knowing I was about to lose my breast did not in any way make me feel lucky. I also thought, yeah, you can say I'm lucky; you are not about to be butchered and deformed."

Natasha S. suggests that when we speak with cancer patients, we never say that things could be worse. Her mother repeatedly used that phrase, and the words didn't help. They only made her feel worse. I don't think one cancer patient would say to another, "It could be worse." Of course it could be. But how does that phrase offer hope?

Micki was to start treatment after her surgery for ovarian cancer. Two cancer survivors tried to give guidance. One downplayed the treatment saying, "Don't worry—no big deal." The other, a nursery school teacher, said she was given treatment on Friday, rested over the weekend, and returned to work on Monday. On the Internet, Micki read of a patient who had trained for the marathon while on chemo. Micki was prepared to "kick ass." A few days before Micki was to start treatment, Regina, a neighbor, dropped by with some lovely gifts of green tea, unscented soap, crackers, and almonds. Regina was subdued, and told Micki that chemo was a "bitch," and Micki faced a really tough road. Regina was not a cancer survivor, so Micki discounted those perceptions. Wasn't she ready to "kick ass?" A week later, Micki was very sick from her treatment. She felt like a failure. She told her husband she was failing as a patient; she was a wimp, a loser, "I was incredibly disheartened," she says.

Ironically, it turned out that Regina's words brought more comfort to Micki than the positive stories had. Yes, Micki commented, the "cheering mattered immensely through the very worst days," but once she realized that chemo *was* a rough road, she could deal with the terrain. Being too positive can be a negative. Patients aren't supermen or superwomen. Cancer doesn't create superheroes; it does create people willing to fight to live.

When I was told how "brave" I was in choosing high-dose chemotherapy and two stem cell transplants to treat my cancer, I felt uncomfortable. Other survivors have told me that they feel the same way when they are told how courageous they are. Yes, it is possible to crawl under the covers and deny the cancer reality; and while at times we all have wanted to do that, actually we have no choice other than just to get on with it. It's not bravery; it's the will to live. Evan Handler, the actor who has since gone on to success in his role in the television show *Sex and the City*, wrote of his cancer struggle in *Time on Fire*. He said, "Running into a burning building when you don't have to, in order to save someone else is brave. . . . I don't see anything courageous about behavior in situations where there is no choice."

Dianne, a two-time cancer survivor, addresses the issue of how being called brave proved a negative rather than a positive. "I felt horrible and sad and totally depressed, and to be repeatedly admired for my strength only made me feel like a fraud, and even more alone and totally misunderstood."

Norman Stanton is a minister and a cancer survivor. I asked him how we, as individuals and as members of a community, can best nurture and support the patient during the cancer struggle. This is his perspective: "I understand that the most important thing I can do for a person who has been diagnosed with cancer is to be a loving presence at what is potentially a very lonely time in a person's life. I want to be supportive of the team of professionals who will be working on specific issues for the person diagnosed as having cancer—doctors, psychotherapists, social workers. In my judgment, my role is not to offer advice or explanations, but to help the person find security in facing what may be ahead for them. . . . One of the special challenges for all caregivers in our time is to help demythologize the word 'cancer,' and help the person who has received that diagnosis to understand that the wonderful advances in medicine in our time have removed that diagnosis from being a 'sentence of death.' "

DECISION TIME

Language cues should always come from the patient. The immediate post-diagnosis period is a particularly difficult time. It is not the time to overload the newly diagnosed person with your ideas, concerns, and recommendations for treatment. A computer system crashes when it is overloaded. Dr. Jimmi Holland states, "Research shows that high anxiety actually makes it harder to process information, just at the time you most need your faculties about you." In your desire to help, don't say or do too much initially. There will be ample time for you to learn what you need to know in order to help.

Be wary about overloading the patient with questions. Not all of them have answers and not all can be answered at the time you ask them. The patients have questions for their medical team, their family, their supervisors, and those from whom they want to ask support. Try not to ask a question that may result in an "I don't know" response from the patient. Unanswerable questions not only create a knowledge gap; they create frustration for the patient. On the other hand, since our role is to create connection, not separation, if we are asked a question and don't know the answer, one appropriate response can be "I don't know, but I'll try to get the information."

"What's your prognosis?" is probably not the best question to ask. To some patients it may sound like "Are you going to live or die?" Even when a doctor prognosticates, he's dealing with averages, possibilities, probabilities—not certainties. I would love to know what my future is, what my prognosis really is. No one can tell me that. No one can tell *you* your prognosis for life. The patient has the right to discuss or not discuss his prognosis with you.

The time will come when you may want to discuss treatment options if the patient or family member raises the issue; but take care not to offer unsolicited advice. You may be eager to help, and indeed, your suggestions may be good ones, but watch out. You wouldn't want your passenger to direct your every move as you drive. This trip is a much more complicated one. If your opinion is valued, your advice may be requested. When you are asked, you can go into an active mode.

Equally important, once decisions are made regarding treatment, avoid the "coulda, woulda, shoulda" comments. Your decision might be different from the one the patient chooses. That doesn't mean your decision would be the better one. Often several options are open to the patient—surgery, surgery plus radiation, chemotherapy, chemotherapy before surgery, chemotherapy after surgery, perhaps just a period of watchful waiting. The list goes on. Even oncologists can disagree on the "best" treatment. Encourage discussion; participate in the discussion if you know the facts, but support the decision once it has been made.

For example, after my breast cancer diagnosis, I had to make decisions regarding treatment. I had already had two transplants and the concomitant heavy-dose chemotherapy. Therefore, my treatment decision required several consultations. In terms of surgery, the basic question was whether I would have the surgery at my community hospital in White Plains or go to a major cancer center such as Memorial Sloan-Kettering or St. Vincent's Comprehensive Cancer Center in New York. I was quite open in asking friends and family their opinions. There were the New York supporters who assumed that the best medical care was available there. "Of course you have to have this done in New York." There were those who respected the fact that an excellent local surgeon was recommended to me, that the White Plains Hospital nurses had known and cared for me over a seven-year period, and that the hospital was only blocks from my home. Follow-up would be relatively easy. I made my decision after a great deal of soul-searching, and had a very positive experience at White Plains Hospital. Those who had pushed for New York supported my decision once I made it.

RESPECT THE PATIENT'S WISHES

In taking your cues from the patient, assume that what is said to you is confidential. Unless you are asked to be the family spokesperson, don't give out information. Ask the patient what he is willing to share. The person undergoing treatment may be quite open about his condition, but don't assume it. In some cases, less and less frequently now, the patient chooses not to reveal his condition to his children. That may not be your style; nevertheless, you have to respect that decision. The issue of how to deal with the diagnosis in a work situation is equally sensitive. Although federal law forbids discrimination, the emotional and physical aspects of the disease may affect office or business interaction. I've known of people who chose to remain silent, fearful of losing clients. There are instances where attitudes at work might be negative rather than positive. You don't want to be the person to reveal a confidence regarding your friend's condition. For example, Michael Korda, a prominent author and editor, was told by a colleague in the publishing world not to speak about his prostate cancer because it could mean the end of his career.

Again, the issue is not what you would do or say, or whether you would share the information with everyone in the office, or what you consider the best treatment option, but what the patient thinks. It is not uncommon, for example, for people to make suggestions to the patient or the caregiver. ("You'll be taking a leave of absence, won't you, while your husband is undergoing treatment?") Generally, if you're asked for your opinion, give it then, but not before. For instance, Julie was diagnosed with stage IV cancer. She and her family are very close. She told her father she was considering going on disability. He advised against it. He thought it would make her less employable when she chose to return to the workplace. The patient initiated the dialog. Because it was she who brought up the topic, it was appropriate that her father give his opinion. Julie has worked throughout her treatment.

DO YOU REALLY WANT TO SAY THAT?

Occasionally someone says, "Everyone is going to die," but I find it objectionable if it's addressed to a person with cancer, even though the statement itself is true. One wouldn't say this to a friend having gall bladder problems or to someone with a kidney stone. Saying it to cancer patients implies that death is more likely. This may be true, but what good comes of saying it? Of course, everyone is going to die. Life is terminal. But we don't and shouldn't live each day in fear of death. No one goes out the door in the morning expecting to be hit by lightning, or struck by a car. Tragedies do happen, as September 11, 2001, made all too evident; yet we cannot lead our lives expecting to be struck down. An etiquette guideline may be, "Do I really need to say this?" We gear ourselves to fill verbal space. Sometimes it is all right to be quiet. Sometimes less can be more.

Are there topics that are off limits? It depends. The most important consideration is how well you know the individual you're talking to. If your relationship goes back years, and if you've often spoken about personal matters, then it's likely that most topics can be discussed. If you did not speak about an individual's sex life, breast size, or baldness before the diagnosis, what makes you think it is appropriate to ask those questions now? The fact that your uncle has prostate cancer doesn't mean he's going to discuss his impotence or catheter problems with you.

Be conscious of the impact your words can have before you bring up certain issues. For example, what is accomplished by saying, "If only you had lost weight," "If only you had exercised more," or "You should have cut down on your red meat"? Cancer hits those who exercise faithfully as well as "couch potatoes." It strikes the fat and the thin. Do diet and exercise improve health? Probably. Is it constructive to imply that the cancer may be his fault? Absolutely not. The man who didn't have regular PSA tests (the Prostate-Specific Antigen test that can indicate prostate cancer), the woman who neglected to have a routine Pap smear (the test that examines cells collected from the cervix), the person who is thirty pounds overweight—they will question their behavior should cancer occur. The classic example is of the individual who develops lung cancer. A common response to this situation is to ask, "Did he smoke?" Suppose he did. He probably knows that smoking contributed to his cancer. These comments may make you feel better because you exercise, you're a vegetarian, and you're not overweight. ("See? It won't happen to me—I do the right things.") But they won't help your mother, your partner, or your best friend as they struggle with cancer reality. This is not the time for an "I told you so" attitude.

A number of years ago, I got a call from someone newly diagnosed with multiple myeloma. He described his condition. I asked what treatment decision he had made. He told me that he had met with a nutritionist who recommended a high carrot diet. He felt comfortable with that recommendation even though his son was unhappy with his decision. What could I say? In truth, I thought he was an idiot. I wished him luck, and told him he could call me at any time. Months later, he did call—from the hospital—and told me how he regretted his decision. His condition had worsened, and he was now getting chemotherapy. Sometimes it is necessary that we keep our opinions to ourselves. This man didn't ask what I thought; he told me what he was doing.

"I KNOW HOW YOU FEEL"

Beware of the "I know how you feel" comment, even if you have dealt with cancer, too. There are more than a hundred types of cancer. New protocols and clinical trials are announced almost daily. Less than ten years ago, research was being done on 124 possible anticancer agents. Now that number has grown to more than 400. Surgical techniques are improved upon routinely. Unless you have had exactly the same cancer, the same stage, the same cell type, the same treatment, it's really not the best thing to say. Selma Schimmel, in *Cancer Talk*, tells of a cancer survivor who said, "I know how you feel" to a young adult. The patient responded, "But now that I've had a hysterectomy, I'm never going to be able to have a child. Maybe you know how I feel physically, but you have no idea what it is that I feel." Every case, every patient is different. How can I compare my situation to the mother whose son has leukemia? The teenager undergoing treatment for non-Hodgkin's lymphoma will probably become sterile. I can't really know how she feels. Except in rare circumstances, saying, "I know how you feel" is just not going to work. "I think I may know how you feel" is a more realistic statement. This may sound picky, but the newly diagnosed patient is vulnerable, and may overreact to ill-considered comments.

Hold the war stories. There's no need to create a situation where there can be verbal overload. Saying, "I had chemo and I was sick for weeks," or "I had VAD and it can really damage your heart" is not helpful to someone contemplating those therapies. Medicines to counter the effects of chemotherapy are now much more effective than they were years ago. Your goal is to give support and strength, not to add to the anxiety level. Some patients vomit just on entering the hospital, so great is their fear.

Keep in mind this question. "Will my story help or hinder?" When in doubt, forget about telling your experience. However, if you have some specific information about a new treatment or protocol, you can ask the patient if she would want material on the topic. The delicate issue is how to present information and experiences without implying that the current medical path is incorrect. You might also ask yourself, "Will the information add to or lessen the patient's stress?"

We are not alone in worrying about what to say and how to say it. Clergy share our concerns. The Reverend Peter Gibbons, a Roman Catholic priest who participated in a clinical pastoral education program at a major medical center, learned what not to say. "I am not going to explain why a God would take a child from a mother. . . . We are trained to be a witness and a presence, and to let them feel they are not alone."

Unfortunately, only some doctors are aware of the importance of what they say. Dr. Jerome Groopman in his most recent book, *The Anatomy of Hope*, discusses the importance of language. He speaks of the M & M conference (for morbidity and mortality) where physicians discuss errors in judgment or technique, issues of critical importance if errors are not to be repeated. Groopman says, "But there was no similar conference about language, no analysis of errors in judgment or technique about what we said to patients and their families." He had been particularly pained about two cases early in his career where he felt words hurt rather than helped. Those cases taught him how powerful words could be, especially if they were the wrong words. "Yet, I still wasn't sure how to speak and what to say."

TOUGH TOPICS

As uncomfortable as it may be, expect difficult topics to be raised. It's better to struggle with an issue than to avoid it. In her book, *Seeing the Crab*, Christina Middlebrook writes of her 16-year old daughter. Maggie was eager to get her driving license. When Maggie failed her driver's test, Christina, even in the midst of chemotherapy, had to continue to chauffeur her daughter around. She thought this might be her daughter's attempt to keep her mother alive. She said, "Talking about my dying, Maggie, is not going to kill me. Not talking about it will not save my life."

Finding a way to talk about the physical and emotional pain of cancer is not easy. The patient wants to protect the family, and the family wants to protect the patient. At times, I've felt that everyone was willing to talk about anything but the possibility that I might die. Try to find the right words that will keep you connected to the person you're concerned about. Any words that mean the patient had better not go "there" may be counterproductive.

If you say, "Don't even think about that," or "I don't want to talk about that," you may shut down communication. It may be your discomfort that prompts the comment, but your discomfort level is not what's important at this time. What is important is what the patient is worrying about, not what your needs are. For example, the issue of death is often on the patient's mind even if the cancer is at an early stage, even if the prognosis looks good, even if the surgery was successful. The cancer patient is afraid of dying. Historically, cancer has been equated with death. If the patient says, "I'm afraid of dying, " or "What will happen to my family if I die?" you have the responsibility to listen and to respond. Saying, "Don't worry; you're not going to die" is not going to help. It denies and demeans the patient's fears. He's raised the most basic of life's questions; do not dismiss him. Talk to him. Handle it as a real possibility.

I've said to someone with metastatic cancer, "I don't want to talk about your dying, because I don't want you to die." It was an honest statement, yet it left the door open for our discussion, and we did talk about death. No one wants to acknowledge the possibility of death. If the patient raises the question with you, directly or indirectly, it means *she* trusts you. If *he* trusts you, you have to participate in the dialog, painful though it may be.

The possibility of death is the monkey on everyone's back. Talking about it at least acknowledges the monkey's presence. If the medical situation is critical, then a professional may need to be called in to bring the issue to the surface. The goal is for you to keep the communication flowing, always taking your cues from the patient.

A young man was dying of cancer, and no one wanted to speak to him about it. After he died, his family found journals in which he spoke of his isolation because no one talked to him about what was happening. The cues were missed.

YOU CAN FIND THE RIGHT WORDS

Sometimes the simplest words are the best. The author, Joseph Telushkin, tells the story of an old man who is at his wife's gravesite. The guests have left, except for the rabbi and the man. The man keeps saying, "I loved my wife." Again and again, the rabbi indicates it's time to leave. Finally, the man says, "But you don't understand. I loved my wife, and once, I almost told her." When a close relative or friend is diagnosed with cancer, possibly the most important statement you can make is, "I love you." It's equally important for the person with cancer to tell those closest to him the same thing. Although my children knew that I loved them, I needed to tell them, again and again. I still tell them in virtually every conversation we have. They do the same. It's amazing how easy it gets, and how meaningful it is.

Children can teach us the importance of admitting the love we have for another. Joel Nathan, in *What To Do When They Say "It's Cancer,"* writes about a mother who told her daughter she had cancer. The child replied, "Don't worry, Mum. I love you like elastic. No matter where you go, it will stretch."

There are no magic words. The magic is that friends and family are generally there for us. Though we may err in our words, we keep trying to do it right. The magic is that we can survive the words "You have cancer," and proceed on a healing path. The magic is that most words do give strength. It's in the invisible connection between two people talking. It takes practice to make magic.

Who would have thought that our language would have improved so much that a play dealing with a professor dying of ovarian cancer could win a Pulitzer Prize, and that audiences would pack the theatre to see it? The play was then made into a successful movie for HBO. We may not have the skill with words that Margaret Edson has in *Wit,* but we can use our words to help those we care about. We can choose our words carefully, and therefore help bring control to a world that is, at least temporarily, out of control. That is the true magic.

4
WHAT WE DO

"If you need me, I'm here." "Anything you want, just call." "How can I help?" We've all made statements like these. But however sincere and heartfelt, they are too general, too amorphous. With what you do as with what you say, the needs will vary as the patient moves from diagnosis to treatment and then survival. The good news is that more and more patients live many years after treatment. Seventy-five years ago, the primary task after a patient was told he or she had cancer was for the family to deal with the likelihood of death. Today, even though the specter of death is never totally erased, most cancer patients survive with a life of high quality. We recognize the dramatic changes in treatment. We've seen the medical breakthroughs. Now, how we react needs to reflect the improved prognosis the patient enjoys.

Just as an IV is a conduit for the drugs that enter our body to destroy cancer cells, just as the IV provides pain relief or transmits antibiotics to kill germs, so, too, the things we do serve as metaphorical IVs during the periods of diagnosis, treatment, and survival. Our words and what we do are as critical to the healing process as any intravenous drug. The positive emotional infusions that promote healing, though not visible, must be monitored just as carefully as the healing infusions on the metal poles found in every hospital room.

Because the cancer calendar often extends for years and years rather than weeks or months, it is essential that caregivers, friends, colleagues, and family act for the long term. A ten-minute visit to the hospital or a lasagna offering is lovely for a neighbor or a casual acquaintance, but it will not suffice for those closely connected to the patient.

STAY CONNECTED

Our mantra should be "Stay with it." Connecting means recognizing that healing takes place on a continuum. Cancer dramatically alters the patient with respect to his or her world of love, work, and friendship. Whatever we do, great or small, that bridges the gap between the patient's worlds of illness and health will be helpful. If Hansel hadn't spread the crumbs, he and Gretel would not have been saved. Your deeds, those seemingly unimportant crumbs, will be important markers on the patient's path back to health.

The importance of your active participation cannot be overestimated. Too many cancer patients talk of the disappearance of friends once a diagnosis is made, or after treatment starts. Later, some make excuses. They were busy. They didn't want to bother the patient. They were too upset to be useful. They couldn't face visiting someone in the hospital. These are unacceptable excuses. Dr. Karen Ritchie calls those who disappear bolters. ". . . their distance reflects their own discomfort. They stay away because they are afraid of their own sadness or their own mortality."

Dr. Lawrence Altman, in a science column in *The New York Times*, reviewed several studies presented at a meeting of the American Society of Clinical Oncology. He reported that a team of doctors under the aegis of Dr. Michael J. Claritz found that married women with brain tumors were eight times more likely to get divorced or separated than men with the same condition. Male doctors were surprised at the findings, but Dr. Glantz noted, ". . . none of the nurses, colleagues and other women I work with was surprised."

This study is a startling example of the fact that sometimes a spouse cannot accept the reality of cancer. The greatest mistake, for anyone, is to disappear from the life of a cancer patient. If it is the spouse, the blow must be devastating. How can it not be felt as rejection? The patient should not have to add that distress to a situation already filled with high anxiety and challenge. The disappearance of a friend, while less traumatic than that of a spouse, is still painful nevertheless. It takes effort and determination to stay connected.

Few of us will consistently know the perfect answers or the perfect responses. There's nothing wrong with saying, "I don't know what to do." However, with some thought, you will be able to say, "Let's talk about what I can do."

The first critical period requiring action occurs immediately after diagnosis, although in some cases, your help will be needed during the shorter pre-diagnosis phase as well. There is much to contribute once a cancer diagnosis is confirmed. One goal is to do nothing that makes the patient feel less of a person, less capable, less able to deal with life, less able to remain in contact with friends and family, just because he or she now has cancer. If you used to talk to your spouse about problems at work, don't stop doing so because she has cancer. If you trusted your friend's judgment when it came to your rebellious daughter, continue talking about your concerns. The patient has cancer. That doesn't mean he or she has lost the ability to listen and still be a vital part of your life.

GETTING THE NEWS OUT

The patient, and everyone in the patient's constellation, is overwhelmed at this first stage. The influx of calls may be excessive, and yet the patient may still want to answer calls personally. You can offer to be an information gatekeeper. Even if the patient is screening his calls, constant repetition of the latest cancer news is enervating. If you take on the role of information ombudsperson, you free the patient and caregiver to focus on the major medical decisions that need to be made. Sometimes more than one information liaison is needed.

When I was diagnosed, I asked two school colleagues to serve as my representatives. The faculty, staff, and administrators called upon them for updates instead of bombarding me with questions. That took care of my professional life; my children did the rest. The information liaison can screen calls, take messages, or return calls.

Today, with the pervasiveness of e-mail, communication is easier than it used to be. E-mail permits virtually instant communication. Your task may be to communicate with others on a daily or weekly basis, depending on the patient's condition or personal wishes.

If a colleague has cancer and is not disclosing it, or is not telling his children, the issue of confidentiality is critical. For those who are open about their diagnosis, if you are in charge of e-mail communication, you can keep family and friends updated on the patient's condition and course of treatment. If you are the e-mail representative at work, be sure to get approval from your supervisor before using the company's computer for this purpose. If there is a sick bank at work, you can volunteer to coordinate the donation of sick days to the patient.

THE INTERNET

There may be a need not only for information gatekeepers but for research coordinators as well. The amount of information about cancer is overwhelming. Patients need information if they are to make informed decisions. What are the most common protocols? What does it mean to be Stage IIb? Where are the major cancer centers located? How does one find a support group? What is a clinical trial? These are only some of the questions you can help to answer. Whatever your role, ask the patient's permission before you act. Rather than handing over a sheaf of papers filled with information from cancer sites on the Internet, ask if it is all right to do some research. Not everyone wants to be immersed in the information whirlpool at the same time, or with the same depth. If information is power, by gathering data and transmitting it in an understandable way, you are extending power to someone who may feel powerless. Large university medical centers have web sites. The Arkansas Cancer Research Center, for example, has several sections, one for self-referral, another for making a first appointment, one for physician's referral, and more. Search the Memorial Sloan-Kettering Cancer Center site and you can find information on cancers, treatments, clinical departments, and physicians, etc. You can even subscribe to a free e-mail newsletter. You can investigate many other relevant sites.

There are caveats in terms of the Internet, however. Is the information from a reliable source? Is it from a medical or academic journal? Have the sites been developed by teaching hospitals or major cancer organizations? Be sure to do your homework and check out the reliability of the sites. If you are handing over information, be certain it is data you can trust. Be sure it is current. The library can be a major resource for those who don't have a computer.

SUPPORT GROUPS

You may want to find information about support groups. You can locate cancer organizations relevant to the patient's condition. The Association of Cancer Online Resources (ACOR) for example, has 133 mailing lists. The subscriptions are free, and one can get information and support for virtually every type of cancer. Patients, caregivers, friends from all over the world communicate, using the lists. Gilda's Clubs provide networking groups for patients, caregivers, and the children of patients. There is access to the American Cancer Society and the Leukemia/Lymphoma Society in many, many communities. Gathering information about support groups, whether they be in the neighborhood or online, can be extraordinarily useful. You may want to wait before offering the information. Support groups aren't for everyone, and not everyone will be ready at the same time. During the diagnosis phase, the patient may be too overwhelmed for a support group. Later on, if he or she raises the issue or asks a question, you will have the information readily available.

Be a go-fer. You can offer to schedule medical appointments for consultations, pick up needed medical documents, provide transportation to and from appointments, or take charge of car pooling, if there are young children involved. Medical equipment may need to be rented. If health care aides will be needed, you can offer to do the interviewing. Volunteer to coordinate these tasks when necessary. There is no end to the possibilities.

PAPERWORK

During this diagnosis period, the patient has to make many critical decisions. Cancer reality requires the patient to deal with issues that many postpone, even when life is normal. If finance or law is your area of expertise, offering support in this arena might be a good choice for you. When I was diagnosed with multiple myeloma, the therapist I consulted was quite definite in telling me to get my affairs in order. I signed a power of attorney, wrote a will, set up a living will, and designated a health care proxy. Most difficult, I purchased a cemetery plot. Doing this may be an extreme measure, but depending on the circumstances, it might be necessary. Even these seemingly depressing decisions can give a sense of control to the patient.

Another task you can volunteer for is to assist with the medical insurance claims and follow-ups. This will reduce the workload and relieve stress on the family. The patient could ask you to track his medical progress on a spreadsheet. This is particularly useful as blood counts rise and fall during the course of treatment.

TAKE OVER

Simple tasks still need to be done. Because I was treated far from home for weeks at a time, I had one friend take care of my mail. I signed checks, and provided stamped envelopes, then left for Little Rock. My friend,

Teddy, paid the bills as they came due. Be prepared for a major commitment if you take on any of these responsibilities. You will be needed until the patient has recovered enough to take the load back.

Having to make decisions alone or in crisis mode simply adds to the difficulty of the patient's situation. Even a simple task, such as obtaining the necessary business forms, will be helpful. During this phase, the cancer etiquette of words and deeds merge. For example, if the patient hasn't discussed any substantive issues, a question may stimulate action. "Have you thought of getting a health proxy?" Again, ask rather than tell. Consider saying to your colleague, friend, or loved one, "When I was sick, I was glad to have a therapist to talk to. If you're interested, I can get you the names of some therapists."

LITTLE THINGS MEAN A LOT

During the diagnosis whirlwind, patients still need to stay connected to the non-cancer world. One of the most difficult challenges I faced, and still do, is to retain my integrity, to remain whole, in spite of the fact that I have been battered and scarred. It's not easy to balance the cancer life with the non-cancer life. Anything you can do that permits the patient to straddle the two is helpful. Ask your friend if he or she wants to go out for dinner, to the movies, shopping. It's one escape from the cancer life, if only temporarily.

Once treatment starts, those opportunities may need to be adjusted to the vagaries of chemotherapy, radiation, or recovery from surgery. However, don't "write off" the patient in any way. If she is too tired, anxious, or depressed, she will decline your invitation. Give her the option. Once again, you're offering to act, yet at the same time you're ceding control to the patient. Lynn Redgrave, the actress, knows how important it is that she have control over her breast cancer. "It's all about order," she decided. During her chemotherapy treatment, Redgrave realized that when she folded napkins and put them into her closet, when she saw to it that the cats were fed, when she took out the garbage—she knew she had some control. One guideline is that we should help the patient find control amidst what may seem like cancer chaos.

Giving the patient "calendar control" helps. Making "play dates" throughout the process is good. Maybe the dates won't always work out, but they need to be scheduled. Why is it that we can schedule business appointments, doctors' appointments, therapists' appointments, but we often find it difficult to schedule pleasure? Continue to schedule the "good stuff" with your friend, colleague, or loved one whenever possible during this period. The "bad stuff" will, of necessity, find its place on the calendar.

JUST BE THERE

One may not even be aware of how significant an action can be. Its importance lies in the heart of the person who feels the link. Ned R. was at a conference when he got the bad news of his wife's diagnosis. He booked the first flight in the morning, having missed the last evening flight. At dinner that night, he told the conference organizers what had happened. One of the co-chairs, a total stranger, "one of the busiest, hardest-working, most sleep-deprived people at the conference," decided Ned shouldn't be alone. She stayed with him as he cleared up his hotel bill, walked with him to the concierge's desk, and rode up in the elevator as he went to his room. With a quick hug, she was gone. Few words were exchanged. Her presence was what counted. Words weren't necessary. Never underestimate the impact of just being there.

When I was told I would lose my hair, I asked a friend to go with me to get fitted for a wig. A young woman was sitting in the area reserved for people needing hair replacement. She was young, pale from treatment; a scarf covered her head. She was probably waiting to pick up a wig that had been washed and styled. Quietly, she said to me, "Don't worry; you'll get used to it." In truth, I never did, but what's important was that she, at that moment, was able to sense my anxiety and respond to it. In spite of where she was, she connected to where I was at that moment.

Your pain as friend, colleague, or family member is real. Nevertheless, your pain needs to be set aside, so that the pain of the patient is eased rather than intensified. In *At the Will of the Body*, Arthur Frank, writing of his cancer experiences, says, "Human suffering becomes bearable when we share it. When we know that someone recognizes our pain, we can let go of it."

The support you give during the diagnosis phase will continue to be needed through the treatment phase, which extends over a longer period of time. New etiquette opportunities will arise. Treatment often starts with hospitalization. The hospital stay is now days rather than weeks. Your first contact with the patient after diagnosis, therefore, may be at the hospital. Your visit can contribute to healing.

VISITING IN THE HOSPITAL

If the patient has had major surgery, the visitors during the first 24 to 48 hours should be the immediate family. However, if the patient is up to it, and encourages visitors, keep the visit brief. Call before you visit. You wouldn't "drop in" at a friend's house without calling; don't do so now. If your friend were at home, and said, "Come on over," you'd still ring the bell before you entered. Knock on the door of the hospital room and ask permission to come in. If he's asleep, tiptoe away, go to the waiting room, or come back at another time. You're being no more courteous than you would be in the non-cancer world; and by asking, you're again giving a sense of control to the patient.

Even if you're a very close friend or relative, don't overstay your visit. Your presence means a lot, but the patient shouldn't feel he has to entertain you. He's tired; she doesn't really want to talk too long. The patient is likely to respond better to visits early in the day. By afternoon, fatigue sets in. If the patient is in intense pain or heavily medicated, the best etiquette may be to wait until the patient goes home. When in doubt, ask.

If there are small children who want to visit a parent, offer to take the kids to and from the hospital. Elderly relatives want to visit; they might need transportation. If you volunteer to do this, you can also monitor the length of the visit. You are eager to cheer your friend, and partying can be a distraction, but your friend is likely to be sharing a room. For a visitor, that means respecting the privacy of the roommate.

Try to avoid what very often happens. A visitor arrives and remains standing at or near the door, giving the impression of appearing to be interested only in escape. Going to see a patient should be by choice, not obligation. Such a visit accomplishes nothing. If you are too uncomfortable to concentrate on the patient, reschedule the time to call.

When the doctor enters the room to examine or talk to the patient, that's your signal to step out. The patient endures many indignities in the hospital. Catheters, tubes, and hospital gowns do little to enhance a person's self-image. You should not be there during any procedure, unless the patient specifically asks you to stay.

Food often serves as a way to share, to connect, even in the hospital. Few look forward to hospital fare. Here's an opportunity for nutritional creativity. Bring snacks or treats to patients in the hospital. Have a "patient picnic." Bring take-out food in, but keep in mind the diet the doctor has ordered. If it's an unrestricted diet, then almost anything goes. Hospital food to many of us is a cut above airplane food, but not by much. Your food contributions will comfort as well as nourish.

VISITING AT HOME

What does the patient need? Where is he or she emotionally and physically at that moment? It's natural during a visit to talk about the patient's physical condition, but conversation that includes news of the everyday world is also good. Telling stories about work, about parties, about movies might make some patients feel isolated, but I think it connects them to their non-cancer world. It reminds them that they will return to that community in time. Don't be afraid to ask advice from your friend, colleague, or parent if you've done so in the past. The fact that he has cancer doesn't mean he has lost his ability to evaluate what you're saying. Obviously, if the patient is sedated or in a weakened condition, you're not likely to get involved in a serious discussion.

Remember the relationship you had before cancer. Doing so reminds the patient that he or she can still make a contribution to your life. The visit then becomes interactive. However, don't do what one young woman did. She was visiting her friend who had had a mastectomy. Sometime during the visit, she directed the conversation to her own planned breast enlargement surgery—an incredibly insensitive thing to do.

With the patient home, you can provide distractions: an afternoon movie, a manicure excursion, or simply a walk. These acts demonstrate that not only will there be life *after* chemotherapy, there is life *during* chemotherapy. The patient may be on a full or partial hiatus from community, from work, from most activities. Do what you can to see that the hiatus isn't an emotional one as well.

If you want to offer help, be specific. Specificity will achieve two goals. First, real needs can be met. For example, "Do you want me to make copies of the pathology reports?" "Can I drive you for your blood tests?" "What time do you want me to be at the house?" "There's a healing service this Thursday at church. Would you care to join me?" I phrase these as questions, not statements, because by asking rather than telling, you are again restoring a sense of control to the patient. Anything that provides a sense of structure and control is likely to be helpful. Telling creates a situation where the weak one, the patient, appears to be responding to the strong one. Asking creates collaboration. Anything that makes the patient feel more of an outsider, more incapable of action and decision, or less in control weakens rather than strengthens.

NOURISHING THE PATIENT

Many things during this period will continue to center on food. Even here, there is a need for organization. If the battle metaphor for cancer is a valid one, then the treatment period requires a quartermaster corps, particularly when it comes to food. Once the patient goes home, there will be issues of shopping, food preparation, cleanup, and family dietary preferences. A food coordinator can assign nights for the "food crew." The meals should be complete, including salad, vegetables, and dessert. If you don't use disposable containers, keep track of casserole dishes. You don't want the patient to worry about whose pot is sitting on top of the stove.

Foods that can be nibbled on are good choices. A pot of meatballs, a batch of chicken wings, a large bowl of tuna fish will last several days. The patient may prefer to have several small snacks, rather than one large meal. If you agree to prepare a meal, cleanup is part of the deal. Instead of saying, "I'm here for you," the better offer would be "Do you want me to cook on Tuesday or Wednesday?" or "Do you prefer roast chicken, or chicken salad?" For variety, give certificates for take-out meals; then the family can choose the menu. If there are young children involved, invite them out for pizza, or for ice cream treats. This is not the time for gourmet meals so keep the food simple.

No matter how hard you try, the person you most want to nourish may not have much of an appetite. For those undergoing chemotherapy, the sight of food, the smell of food, even the thought of food is repugnant at times. Many patients have a metallic taste in their mouths, or dry mouth, which overpowers normal taste sensations. Mouth sores or thrush affect both appetite and taste. In many instances, therefore, the concept of three balanced meals must be scrapped. Whatever the patient craves, whatever tastes good, whatever works (with the doctor's approval) should be provided. Some patients need nutritional supplements. If you have a recipe for a homemade shake, make it and see if it satisfies the patient. The husband of one patient bought a juice machine. He has become a "master juicer" and creates exotic juices every day. If you're cooking a casserole, in some cases it will be useful to divide it into individual resealable serving dishes. This helps if the family doesn't eat together and, since the patient may eat small servings at odd times of the day, individual portions may prove more efficient.

Be imaginative about food. If your wife wants ice cream for breakfast, I'd say go for it. When will she be able to do that again without caloric guilt? There are likely to be idiosyncratic elements to what the patient craves or can eat during the treatment period. I didn't eat well for months. At one point, I had a craving for Genoa salami, and managed to keep that down. It sounds odd that I could eat what is too spicy for many healthy people. The spices were strong enough to take away the metallic sense. An Irish member of our support group craved chicken noodle soup with matzoh balls during her treatment. I remember her joy when I brought a large pot of soup for her.

In another instance, a passion for oysters brought pleasure to a patient. Dick brought fresh oysters to Richie's house several times a week. It was one of the few foods Richie could tolerate. Who would have thought a gift of oysters could be so treasured? Offer the offbeat food choice; you never know what might stimulate the patient's appetite. However, if there are very unusual cravings, such as an excessive urge for sweets, or salt, check with the doctor.

Ruth H. knows the importance of the connection food can bring. She started baking banana muffins for her neighbor who had cancer of the larynx. Remission was short-lived. Because a feeding tube became necessary, she could no longer eat the muffins. But her husband, the primary caregiver, still needed the muffins for *his* emotional nourishment. Ruth started adding cranberries and calling them "get well pills." She included a card with the muffins, telling her friend that the prescription could be renewed at any time, with no charge for delivery. Later on, Ruth continued baking the muffins for the family. It's no surprise that through the ages, food has been a way of connecting.

Snacks are good. The patient whose appetite is poor might be tempted by sweets. Candy kisses are great; they even send a message, and somehow, chocolate soothes. For non-chocolate lovers, there are other treats such as ice cream, Popsicles, or yogurt. For some, pretzels or chips work, but first determine whether there is a salt restriction. A homemade soup is nutritious and relatively easy to digest. Never underestimate the comfort of a good soup. Cancer patients are encouraged to drink lots of liquids; soup counts as one. You may want to go to a gourmet shop or, in season, to a farm stand to buy homemade preserves. Try buying an exotic coffee or a variety of teas. In winter, hot chocolate is good. A variety of hard candies can also negate the effects of dry mouth.

In some instances during treatment, fresh fruits, salads, and raw vegetables will be forbidden. If a patient's white blood count is too low, the patient is susceptible to infection, thus the prohibition. This temporary condition is called *neutrapenia*. The patient has little resistance to infection at this time. Bacteria in fresh food or vegetables could be dangerous; therefore, check with the doctor before you bring in certain foods and fresh flowers.

5 GIFTS OF MANY KINDS

What's a good gift? Can there be an incorrect gift? A boyfriend's mother visited the hospital and gave the young woman patient a sheer, sexy nightgown. Not the right choice, at that time, for someone being treated for breast cancer. There are probably a few such gift gaffes, but thankfully not too many. Still, some gifts are better than others. Just as the right words can make the patient feel he or she is linked to the real as well as the cancer world, so too can personal gifts. A bottle of moisturizer, for example, is not only good for a woman's skin, often dry from chemotherapy, it serves as a reminder that she is still a woman. Bath oils last, and a warm bath can be a great way to help someone to relax. Perfume is less likely to be a good idea because one's sense of smell is often affected by treatment. Bedclothes that button in the front will be better than those that go over the head. Women who have had breast surgery cannot easily raise their arms, and any patient with a chest catheter will prefer garments that open in the front.

For a man, an electric razor will be a practical gift. A man using an electric shaver is less likely to get a cut that can become infected. After-shave lotion is a good gift, but avoid too strong a scent if someone is undergoing chemotherapy. Men also enjoy clean-scented soaps as well as soothing skin lotions. Gifts of "promissory notes" work. Promise to babysit. Volunteer to weed the garden for a month. Tape your friend's favorite television shows.

Gift certificates are also welcome. How about one for a manicure and a pedicure? A homeowner might welcome a certificate for Home Depot, the golfer one at the local sports shop. Yoga lessons can help the patient recuperate. A gift for rental movies is great for when it is not feasible for the patient to go out. Since there is usually no time limit on gifts of this type, the patient can sign up once he or she gets the doctor's approval. A gift certificate for dinner for two in a restaurant, a day at the spa, theater tickets, serve as reminders that at some point patients will heal and resume their roles as wives, husbands, lovers, friends, colleagues, parents, grandparents, and members of a community.

Books are a favorite as gifts. Still, think about your selection. Patients having heavy-duty chemo are not likely to read heavy-duty books. Some patients welcome books about those who have achieved remission; others do not want to read about some one else's cancer. Cheryl T. was thrilled to get two books as gifts. One was on breast cancer, because that's what she was going through, the other on ceramics because "that's who I am." Because it was her best friend who gave her the books, she could accept the fact that the friend knew she needed both information and recognition that she still had interests other than cancer.

Books that proselytize or speak about how God will heal might not be appropriate for everyone. If the person is devout, religion as a topic is a possibility. If you don't know the patient's religious leanings, go to another section in the bookstore. Be careful of books that deal with alternative medicine, because you don't want to suggest, however subtly, that patients think of a different kind of medical treatment in lieu of what has already been prescribed for them. You don't know whether the patient wants to go in that direction at this time. Later, if you learn that the patient is interested in books on guided imagery, meditation, biofeedback, or other aspects of complementary medicine, you may consider those topics as options. Books on tape and videotapes are also good gifts, as are compact discs.

The value of humor is well known, so you are not likely to go wrong if you choose humor as a subject. Silly videos can be terrific. Consider a magazine subscription. It can bring weeks or months of pleasure. If your friend did a great deal of traveling, a travel magazine may or may not work. If it serves as a reminder of what the patient will be able to do, then it may be a good choice. If the idea of travel is not a realistic one, it can cause angst rather than pleasure. Offering a choice to the patient or caregiver might work. "I'm going to order a gift subscription. Would Bob like a magazine on current affairs or tennis?" Someone who doesn't have the energy to concentrate on a book might be able to focus on an article. Subscriptions can be a good gift for the children of an ill parent. Magazines appeal to children, and can serve as a distraction for them as well.

I found that chemotherapy definitely affected my powers of concentration. Listening or watching was less taxing than reading. Try to sense what the patient needs, not what you might want to give. Even with gifts, you can ask. "I'm going to the book store. Is there a title you want me to pick up?" "Steve Martin wrote a new book. Would you want to read it?" Crossword puzzles are good if the patient's concentration level is returning. The same is true of jigsaw puzzles. Playing cards are great diversions. Solitaire, double solitaire, rummy, blackjack for pennies—all serve to pass time and engage the patient. Some find that board games help pass the hours. If the patient spends a good deal of time in bed, a lap desk or book lamp can be a good choice. If she will be hospitalized for a while, get a composite picture frame and let her fill it with favorite snapshots. For computer buffs, a game works. Even today, when I need distraction, I'll play solitaire or video poker on my computer. Game discs are not expensive but you need to know the type of computer to make certain the game is compatible with the patient's machine.

If you are a computer surfer, consider giving a gift of a list of web sites for a patient who's a neophyte. For example, if someone is interested in ancient history, search cave drawings. Create a list of museum sites. Give a gift of a CD of a museum's collection. When your friend is up to it, he can visit the museum via his computer.

The patient will be receiving many gifts. How about a box of thank-you notes or a new pen? Be sure to include stamps. You may consider several small gifts rather than one large one. Michelle H.'s sister is a nurse in an ICU. She brought a care package that included wine, chocolate, and Lysol! That's quite a combination. Michelle's gift is successful because it reflects the fact that her sister knows her tastes, and it acknowledges the reality that everyone has to be careful about not spreading germs. A gift of sterile wipes can be a good one. That way, visitors can quickly wash their hands, lessening the chance for infection.

Small gifts mean you will always have something to give. One possibility is a sleep mask. A mask is inexpensive but will be very useful to someone who has difficulty sleeping in the hospital or at home. At a crafts fair or in a department store, you might spot a coffee mug or scarf that will bring a dash of color to the patient's life. Buy socks. Patients often feel cold. Socks in jazzy colors or wild designs will provide warmth and perhaps a laugh as well. Another small gift that can be fun is a few instant lottery tickets. The patient can scratch the cards to look for a win. What a delightful irony for a cancer patient to collect lottery money!

Many cancer patients keep a journal, in part to keep track of their medical progress, but often to record their feelings. If someone expresses an interest in writing, ask if he would like the gift of a journal. For those who want to remember their experiences, but not to write about them, consider giving a tape recorder. Speaking even privately may relieve stress for some.

THE DOLPHIN

Even the smallest gift can be meaningful. During my treatment for myeloma, I had a nightmare. I dreamed I was in a boat, fishing. Suddenly a shark came charging toward me. There was no question he would hit me directly. But instead of being crushed by the shark, I found myself riding to safety on the back of a dolphin. I told the story to a friend. We agreed the dream was a tale of survival. Weeks later, shortly before Easter, Judy M. was in a supermarket. The shelves were crammed with chocolate eggs, and stuffed animals, chicks and rabbits. Mixed in with the Easter items was one lone dolphin. Judy decided that was my dolphin. She bought it for me, and I still look at it every day, a reminder of dreams that can come true. Never underestimate the value of a stuffed animal, no matter the age of the patient.

Get-well cards are really a form of gift. They are always welcome; keep sending them. One won't do. Add a few words to the card. Just a signature might give the impression that the task was simply to get the card, sign it, and get it mailed. Taking the time to add a personal note adds dimension to your gesture, which becomes an act of will rather than an obligation.

The cancer online list I subscribe to has more than 1,000 members. E-mails come from around the globe. Most of us will never meet each other, but we share medical information, moments of medical success, our own stories. Recently, Steve, a patient from Australia, had a setback and went to the hospital. A friend from the list suggested we send get-well cards to him. There's nothing unusual about a get-well card, but imagine getting cards from Italy, Israel, and just about every state in the United States. We needed to learn the cost of postage from the United States to Australia. Many sent cards, and they gave Steve "Down Under" a sense of being cared about during a difficult time.

Some people prefer to use e-mail instead of traditional cards. E-mail can supplement cards. It should not replace them, unless that is the only option available. You can send interesting articles, reviews, or jokes via e-mail. These are some of the advantages to e-mail. Patients can read the mail when up to it, and then respond or not. Be sure, however, not to use e-mail as a substitute for your presence during the treatment period. Being there remains important. Don't be a no-show. Your absence will be remembered, as clearly as your presence is.

If you're a craftsperson or an artist, a handmade gift will be very special. Rhoda's niece has breast cancer. In additional to traditional medicine, her niece was using meditation, imaging, and exercise in an effort to fight the disease, and to find "her inner child." Rhoda, an artisan, an expert fabric dyer, and a marvelous seamstress, wanted to give her niece a special gift, so she designed a vest. She used colors she had dyed herself, hues she thought matched her niece's personality. She used pieces of embroidered fabric that had belonged to her niece's great aunt for part of the lining. The vest was a work of art, a labor of love, a priceless gift.

A water colorist, Eloise J., decided to paint something for her friend who had colon cancer. Instead of one picture, Eloise drew small postcard-size watercolors, at least two or three a week, and mailed them to Cynthia. The colors, the beauty of the cards, the connection they provided were a wonderful gift. What made it even more special was its effect on the family. They mounted the cards on a large board so everyone visiting could see them. The beautiful paintings were a splash of color, a splash of life in this sick woman's world.

If you're a carpenter, craft something for your buddy. If you're a sculptor, carve a gift. If you write limericks or poetry, give the gift of words. Gene K. writes poems for special occasions. His web site offers the service without charge. He now adds a note indicating that those who wish to can make a donation to the Multiple Myeloma Research Foundation. Commission a work; honor your patient with a quilt, a sweater, a fishing jacket with hand-tied flies.

Take care when you offer a gift. Occasionally, you might succeed and fail almost simultaneously. A member of Shelly T.'s writing group was undergoing chemotherapy. Shelly asked the group to submit samples of their writing. She then filled a scrapbook with their work, added watercolor artwork to the book, and presented it to Lorna M. as a gift from the group. Lorna was overwhelmed, brought to tears, and yet she managed to write a thank-you note in verse for the group. It was at this point that Shelly failed. She wanted to visit Lorna, who explained that, for the moment, she felt she needed to rest, and preferred to communicate with friends via e-mail. Shelly should have said, "Of course I understand; I'll call next week and if you're up to it, I'll visit then." Instead Shelly said, "I hope you're not depressed or isolating." These are not terrible words, but they weren't the right ones for Lorna at that time. The gift worked; the words failed.

Not all of us are artists, like Domenic Guastaferro. He is an opera singer who gives concerts in his wife's honor and contributes the proceeds to fight cancer. Still, we can create gifts. Instead of a pasta party, have a poster party. People can write notes, create a cartoon, paste a snapshot. Others can do a collage, cutting letters or phrases out of newspapers and magazines. The collage can include scenes of the patient's favorite activities. Children love to paint and draw. Encourage them to make cards and pictures. They can draw a favorite scene, a pet, anything that they think will bring cheer to the patient. You can combine this project with a gift for the children. They never have enough Magic Markers or drawing paper.

NO GIFT WRAPPING NECESSARY

One of the most beautiful gifts I learned about was unwrapped, and it was never handed to the cancer patient. It was visible only once. Russ M. was diagnosed with cancer when he was 38. He and his wife Janelle have five children. They decided at the time of diagnosis that "we wouldn't waste our time together crying about what might happen, or about time we might not have. . . . We said we would dance until we couldn't anymore." Well, one of their sons gave them a moment of "dance" and he didn't even know it.

Russ is an assistant coach for his oldest son's football team. Even Matt's mother admits that their son is big, husky, and SLOW. During one game, Matt intercepted a pass and started lumbering toward the endzone. Janelle writes, "As long as I live, I will never forget the sight of that boy running down the field, with his Dad matching him step for step down the sidelines screaming, 'RUN RUN RUN' . . . or seeing the hug they shared in the endzone, or seeing those two identical sets of green eyes searching me out in the stands . . . or the two grins that stretched the whole field." Father and son had created a football memory, a gift that will never wear out. "No big deal," you might say. However, this father, this dad fighting cancer, didn't say to himself that day, "Hey, maybe I shouldn't run down the field." On that field, for those few moments, cancer did not exist. Can a football interception be a gift? In this case it certainly was.

There are other gifts as well. A donation of blood or platelets literally can give life. Think of it. You're giving the gift of life in exchange for the poisons the patient is getting. Donating money in honor of your friend, colleague, or loved one is always a good idea. A contribution to the hospital in honor of the nursing staff worked well for me. The nurses posted the letter at their workstation. Similar gifts can be made to honor doctors who have truly connected with the patient.

Never underestimate your own individual power. You can give the gift of political clout. Find out about research funding. Contact your senator and congressperson, and pressure them to support legislation for cancer research.

Jana B. found an unusual way to give a gift. She picks up what she calls "lucky money." In one year, by walking and looking, she banked $250. She keeps a separate account, and over the years raised over $1,000 for cancer research just by picking up the loose change others have dropped. Many have found that becoming active in a local cancer organization is a powerful demonstration of how much the individual means to you.

Use your own abilities. Even a foot massage is welcome. Some patients enjoy being read to. It could be poetry, a novel, a humorous book. In this instance, it may not be a bad sign if the patient drifts off to sleep while you're reading.

A ride to the market can be a gift. Laurie P. had just come home after surgery for lung cancer. Within a day, she said she wanted to go to the store so she could select the produce and salads she wanted. It was a small store; she didn't have to wander through aisles and aisles. I could have done the marketing for her, but that half-hour away from home was important to her. It proved that she was regaining control. Within a few days, we started walking together, a few minutes at first. Eventually, she was able to walk three miles. The walking was good for her health, and it was further proof she could "come back."

You don't have to pore through a catalog to give gifts of time. Yet time has great value. Keep in mind that what is most important is the need of the patient on a particular day, at a particular moment. The etiquette is in how you respond to that need. Give your time consistently, especially to the family with young children. Instead of saying, "If you need a baby sitter, call me," try, "I'm taking my kids to the movies on Saturday; can Danny join us?" or "Do you think Sam would like to go to the story hour at the library?" Volunteer to set up carpool schedules for at least two weeks at a time. Doing so will relieve stress for both patient and caregiver. If changes have to be made, you will be responsible for adjusting the schedule. Remember that the radiation and/or chemotherapy will have an impact on the patient and family for months. You will be needed during that entire time. Do it only if you understand the responsibility and are prepared to follow through.

Kukla B. chose to go to her radiation treatments in Manhattan by herself. The trip was at least an hour each way. The treatment itself didn't take long. What better way for her to unwind and prepare for the trip home than to browse through the stores and, when the urge hit, make a purchase? Kukla calls it retail therapy. Since radiation takes many weeks, there may be a time when she will want company. Ask the patient first if he wants company. Afterward, if your friend is too tired to walk or shop, try lunch in a decent restaurant. Help transform the radiation experience into a positive memory.

If the physician approves of the patient venturing to public places, offer cinema therapy if the patient is physically up to it. In the theater, no one can see the pallor of the patient. No one is likely to notice a turban or the fact that the baseball cap doesn't quite hide the baldness. Movies can offer a welcome distraction. Through the magic of film, you can transport the patient away from the cancer world for at least a few hours.

There are no unimportant gifts. There are no unimportant acts. Some may be less romantic than others. Shopping still needs to be done. The refrigerator needs to be cleaned as well as filled. What's lurking on the back shelves? What's growing moldy in the vegetable bin? A clean refrigerator will also mean one less place for germs to grow. Floors must be mopped. If there are dishes in the sink, wash them. Laundry piles up. Clothes still need to be dry-cleaned. There are carpools to maintain. Plants must be watered. Lawns need to be mowed. Library books have to be found and returned. Who's taking the dog to the vet? Who's helping the children with their homework?

Whatever chore you volunteer for, keep your word. Canceling an appointment at the last minute does minor damage when one is well; the damage is more serious when someone is medically overwhelmed and you don't deliver on a promise. The patient is on physical and mental overload. I know I spent so much time trying to cope that I had little space for complications. Yours could be a minor goof, but the patient may perceive it as a much bigger issue. Cancer and its treatment exacerbate patients' reactions.

Whatever your "assignment," consider it your direct connection to the healing process. Years after I was first diagnosed, I can still remember virtually everyone who was there for me, and the very few who were not.

WHERE CHILDREN ARE CONCERNED

A school community can rally, especially if a student is involved. It is not uncommon, for example, for groups of students, generally high school boys, to shave their heads when one of their peers loses his hair during chemotherapy. Instead of the boy with cancer becoming isolated, he becomes part of the "no hair" community at school. In one preschool, the parents rallied for a young teacher who had been diagnosed with breast cancer. She was single and had little family in the area. The parents set up a schedule so that Betsy had someone to drive her to and from every radiation treatment.

The school community can be a very positive force. Cancer is a reality for too many children. The school that accepts that reality, that helps the student to develop coping skills, that is proactive toward the student—this is the school that reduces the student's stress and anxiety. Ann was in high school when her brother died. She channeled some of her pain into creating a resource guide for children who have a family member with cancer. Among her many recommendations were for offers of tutoring, homework assistance, and guidance with college applications. Some schools sponsor swimathons, where students raise money for cancer causes. Youngsters get pledges for every lap that they swim. One student said that while swimming, she really did think of her classmate who was ill. Car washes, too, are good fund-raisers for teenagers.

Taylor is 11 years old and has bone cancer. When Jill, a good friend of Taylor's mom, learned about the diagnosis, she wanted to do something productive for this vibrant young girl, her family, and the community. Jill had an idea. Realizing that 11-year-olds care about how they look, she decided to create a nonprofit company that would sell hair accessories, and key chains. She wanted to channel Taylor's interest into something positive. Jill called on a friend in the hair accessory business who agreed to deal with manufacturing issues. Jill would handle sales. It turned out that Taylor had a gift for design, and became actively involved in the project.

Within a few months, they added belts, wrist and headbands, jewelry, and hats to the line. Within eight months, Tay-Bandz had raised over $100,000. The company, created by Taylor's family and friends, directs the money for pediatric cancer education and research. This is creative synergy, a win-win situation. Taylor can step outside of the cancer box; the phalanx of friends are proactive. In Taylor's words, "Tay-Bandz helped me help others in my situation. It made me feel good that other people could benefit from my suffering—" wise words from a youngster undergoing very difficult treatment.

Louise Albert writes fiction for young adults. She is also a cancer survivor. Her novel, *Less Than Perfect*, deals with typical adolescent issues. Albert uses her own experiences with cancer as it affected her own daughter and the rest of the family.

Laura, the daughter, learns early in the story that her mother has breast cancer. At one point, the mother sits down with Laura and speaks with her, one adult to another. She uses terms such as lumpectomy, mastectomy, node, and radiation. The mother admits her own fears and speaks of the unpredictability of life. Laura offers solace. In this conversation, Laura is not treated as a child. The threat of cancer has almost instantly changed the dynamics of the relationship between mother and daughter. After her mastectomy, the mother attempts to initiate a conversation with her daughter. Laura gives an excuse, saying she has to study for a test. Albert is realistic here. There will be times when adults are willing to talk about the situation, and times when they deny reality. The same is true for adolescents. Cancer overload can hit anyone.

One evening, there is an argument between brother and sister about whose turn it is to clean up. The mother "loses it," and starts screaming about how self-centered her children are. This, too, is reality. Children argue about chores. Someone in chemotherapy will be emotionally frayed. Laura is angry at what's happening to her mother. Cancer is tearing their lives apart.

In a revealing section, Laura and her mother go to a support session for mothers and daughters. When one mother praises her daughter's efforts, Laura is ready to leave. The next mother, however, claims her daughter doesn't support her enough. A third woman says that if there had been a support group for her when her mother had cancer, she wouldn't have been so angry and fearful. She was angry because she didn't want her mother to have cancer and possibly die, and fearful of having breast cancer herself when she was an adult. As a result, she had a hard time treating her mother, whom she loved dearly, in a loving way. When her mother died, she was overcome with guilt for many years.

Hearing these comments has a profound effect on Laura. She realizes that in many ways she had been like this woman, and how awful life would be for her without her mother.

Albert touches on the important issues: getting infor disease; going for a consultation; talking to the children punches. Parents as well as children can be afraid; teenagers will still be teenagers. They can rise to the occasion sometimes, and act like children at other times. We need to pay attention to their special needs.

THE POWER OF COMMUNITY

Community reminds the patient that he is not alone. Wayne's story illustrates the power of community. Wayne is pastor of a small country church. He took a leave of absence during his treatment, which included a stem cell transplant. During treatment, he had to wear a mask because his immune system was compromised and wearing a mask lessened the possibility of infection. One Sunday, he and his wife went to services. They deliberately came to church late, so congregants would not hug him. They planned to sit off by themselves to minimize their direct contact with members of the congregation. The choir was singing as they entered the church. As Wayne and his wife entered, the leader of the choir gave a signal, and everyone put on a mask. The service continued. That's community.

Janet's birthday occurred during her treatment. Her community of sisters and friends had a flowerbed planting party for her. They planted a rose garden, perennials, and annuals. That community created a thing of beauty that will last. They gave their time, their love, their sweat. A labor of love, one might say. By the way, if the patient is in the hospital and you bring flowers from a garden or florist, remember to bring a vase as well.

Ruth G. had cancer and was recovering from surgery. She decided to plan an afghan. She wanted each square to be unique, so she wrote out all 100 patterns on 3x5 index cards. During the next two years, she completed about half of the project. However, her weakness curtailed her efforts. Her husband, David, tried to return the unused yarn, but because it was over six months after purchase, the store would not accept it, a problem of dye lots.

He enlisted the help of his religious community. The result was that a number of congregants spent months completing the afghan. Ruth's imagination and her craft live on in the beautiful afghan that decorates their home. There are two dedications here. Clearly, one is the completion of afghan. However, David knew how important the project was to his .vife. It was his sensitivity that enabled the project to go forward. He is in the afghan as surely as Ruth and the women in the community who worked on it. The Reverend James Conlon recognizes the symbolism of such a project. Quoted in Dick Ryan's book, *Straight from the Heart*, he says, "Building community is like making a quilt: we all have our own patch; yet a common thread unites us."

Sometimes it takes a community to remind an individual of his worth. Dr. Naomi Rachel Remen writes of a patient who had metastatic cancer. The patient, George, felt that except for making money, his life had had no value. With Dr. Remen's permission, George met Stephanie, another patient whose quality of life had been profoundly improved because of the medical device George had manufactured. She invited George to her house, where he met her friends, neighbors, and relatives, all of whom wanted to honor the man who had given her her life back. George had manufactured about 10,000 of the devices, but never made the link between his work and its impact on others. Stephanie, in gathering her community, contributed to George's healing and self-esteem.

Community can exist on the Internet. One story concerns strangers who, via the Internet, gave a gift to someone they had never met. On a cancer list, patients receive daily e-mails. The patients, and often their caregivers, describe treatment, discuss symptoms, ask questions, and speak of their feelings. Hank was on one such list. He spoke of his wife, who was in hospice. He wrote a poem that to some sounded like a suicide note. No one had met Hank; no one knew where he lived. Nevertheless, some stalwart members of the list did their research. They contacted police who were able to locate him and arrange for medical attention. Hank was sedated, and when he awoke, a physician convinced him that his wife still needed him. Hank still participates on the list, offering support to others.

Lisa's community in Asheboro, North Carolina, raised more than $573,000 for the American Cancer Society's annual Relay for Life. Twelve thousand people attended. Five hundred survivors honored the community by walking the first lap. Such fundraisers require intense team efforts. More than 3,300 communities and eight foreign countries have these relays. Whether they are walks, marathons, or concerts, these types of events illustrate the power of community and the power of love. The T-shirts, sweatshirts, pins, and ribbons not only raise money but also serve as visual reminders of commitment to the cause and to the friend.

Community can be large or as small as the members of a book club. My book club has only six members. When I was first diagnosed with cancer, they bought me a portable CD player, a relatively new electronic device in 1993. I took it with me to Little Rock with a supply of classical music. That music sustained me during some very difficult times.

Community exists even in Antarctica. Jerri Nielsen, a physician, and the author of *Ice Bound*, was stationed there when she found a lump and diagnosed her own breast cancer. Using ice cubes as a topical anesthetic, she performed biopsies on herself. In the darkest time of her life, at the darkest spot on Earth, she still remained connected. Her community was there for her. She worked during her treatment; she caroused with her teammates at their parties and feasts. She never lost sight of the micro and macro elements that bring joy. She was thrilled when she had fresh fruit for the first time in months. Lettuce was a treasure to her, as was a knitted hat a friend gave her. In the darkness of the long winter night there, she was still actively immersed in life.

We are more familiar with office communities; they can be very important. In spite of cancer, Judy F. has continued to work. She shops, cooks, and takes care of her family. At the one-year anniversary of her diagnosis, her colleagues created a beautiful scrapbook and filled it with notes and cards. Many also gave her their own little personal treasures— shells, stones, a Kennedy half-dollar. Judy F. calls them her talismans. She mounted them in an old typesetting frame. Every day when she enters her office, she can see those tokens of love. Together, a community and the patient created a treasure, a treasure to share.

A community of music lovers joined to raise more than $250,000 for research at a benefit in Carnegie Hall. The violinist, Joan Kwuon, had discovered a lump in her breast just as she was preparing to be a soloist at the Tanglewood music festival. She was only 30 years old. She began treatment, and later helped found Artists for Breast Cancer Survival. At the end of the concert, Mandy Patinkin, the host, asked breast cancer survivors to rise. Then those who had had a family member who had breast cancer stood. Finally, those who had a close friend with breast cancer also rose. Very few remained seated.

Community can be a strong force for good. Dolly came to work in Janet H.'s home as an au pair. Janet has four sons, two of whom were infant twins. Over the months, she and Dolly became very close; it was a perfect fit. During this time, Dolly developed health problems, including arm pain. Not wanting to be intrusive, Janet didn't ask too many questions. When Dolly's ache turned out to be a malignancy, Janet called a friend, a medical director at a large hospital. He agreed to treat Dolly. Hospital administrators helped Dolly obtain Medicaid benefits, and the doctors accepted assignment for her case.

Dolly seemed to recover, but ultimately the cancer spread. Janet knew that Dolly had two children living in Africa. Aware of how important it was for Dolly to see her children, Janet asked her congressperson for help. When nothing happened, she contacted the representative from Dolly's election district. Still, nothing happened. The doctors wrote to the foreign embassy explaining Dolly's plight. Again, nothing.

Undeterred, the medical director called the U.S. Ambassador to the country in question. The secretary, taking the call, hearing it was a physician who wanted to reach the Ambassador, gave him the hotel phone number where she was vacationing. He reached the Ambassador in her room, and she responded sympathetically to the plight of this young woman who wanted only to see her children. The Ambassador arranged for visas, and a month later, the children arrived in the United States. The medical outcome was negative, but we cannot overstate the salutary effects of the efforts of one individual and the medical community.

Community can be a moving educational force as well. In an effort to encourage black women to have breast cancer screenings, the Arthur Ashe Institute for Urban Health has initiated a program in about 25 beauty salons in Brooklyn. The Institute supplies the salons with plastic breast models, complete with lumps. By examining the models, women get a better sense of what self-examination is, and are motivated to perform the exercise.

Now, in addition to talking about their personal lives, customers talk openly about breast cancer. The women learn together. One woman, Mary P. Green, told another, "Don't forget to check your armpits, too, and look for changes in color." Eventually, Institute trainers will teach barbers how to talk to men about prostate cancer.

Thomas Merton, the renowned Trappist monk, had the ability to see the link between compassion and community. In terms of the parallels between Oriental mysticism and Western tradition, he wrote, "The whole idea of compassion, which is central to Mahayana Buddhism, is based on a keen awareness of the interdependence of all these living beings, which are all part of one another and all involved in one another."

OTHER KINDS OF GIFTS/THE GIFT OF TOUCH

Some of the most precious gifts are intangible; they require no charge card. One such gift is the gift of touch. When we first see the person we care about, a hug may be just what is needed. If this is a dear friend or family member, the hug can come even before the words. If you haven't had a particularly close relationship with the person, asking, "Can I give you a hug?" is a good idea. Later on, as treatment intensifies, especially if the patient's blood counts are low, it's best for everyone to ask for "hug" permission, with consideration to warding off infection.

Not so long ago, someone I knew was in a coma. When I visited, I wasn't sure how I would react, or what I should do. Yet it seemed natural for me to kiss June's forehead, and simply stroke her hair. I hadn't expected it to be so easy to do. Touch provides the literal connection too often missing in our lives. However, use your judgment. Not everyone is comfortable being touched.

What we say to someone whose treatment seems to be effective may be different from what we say to someone whose cancer has metastasized. "How are you doing?" seems ridiculously inadequate in the latter case. Just being with the patient, not words, may be what is needed. Years ago, I visited Abe, who was ill with pancreatic cancer. We had trained for marathons together. He had been in great shape. Shortly after taking early retirement, Abe became ill. When I last visited, he was sitting huddled under a blanket. There was nothing I could say. I sat next to him, rubbing his back and shoulders. He didn't speak, but it was a special visit.

SEEING IS BELIEVING

You ordinarily would not consider eye contact a gift, but it is. When you're visiting, look directly at the patient. Yes, it's OK to water the flowers in the room, to straighten out the serving table, or wipe the kitchen counter, but the primary purpose of your visit is to be there, and being there means just that. It means concentrating on the person you care about. When you look eye to eye, your ability to listen is enhanced. Too often we hear, but we don't listen. What is the patient saying to you? What issues is he willing to talk about? If certain issues aren't being raised, should you ask a leading question? Are you talking too much about yourself?

MOTIVATION

There is another gift that can be quite meaningful. My diagnoses of multiple myeloma and breast cancer came about as a result of routine examinations. Often I ask friends when they had their last mammography or physical. Their following up is a gift for both of us. When I told my hairdresser I was going to have breast surgery, she was concerned and sympathetic. I asked her when she'd had her last mammography; she had never had one. Carol is probably in her forties. Months later, I asked again, but she still had not been tested. She was too afraid. During a recent visit, Carol requested the name and phone number of my gynecologist. Progress.

THE GIFT OF CARE

Never underestimate the value of what you do. After my double mastectomy, my surgeon insisted I have someone stay with me after I was discharged. We negotiated and I finally agreed to three nights. Later, I cancelled the third night unilaterally. Nevertheless, when I came home I did need help. I could not wash my hair because I couldn't easily lift my arms, and I was not allowed to shower. Using the kitchen sink, my friend, Marilyn, washed my hair. I, who always had—and still have—difficulty asking anyone for anything, feel grateful for that moment of care.

As you participate in the patient's cancer life, don't worry so much about what you will say or do that you become immobile. Listen to your voice. Go with your strengths. Go with your heart, but go. It's better to do, than to do nothing, or to disappear. Everywhere on the cancer path, someone can help. Everything we do has repercussions.

THE GIFT OF PRIVACY

At times during all phases of illness, the patient may need some emotional as well as physical privacy. Although connection is a motif of this book, one can still connect without literally being present. At times I need to be alone. Those quiet moments give me the chance to feel what I feel. I don't have to be the good patient, the optimist, the courageous one. Alone, I don't have to be a cancer performer. I can be a woman who's had cancer twice. That's the reality I see every time I look in the mirror, every time my body says, "Stop," and I have to lie down. The presence of cancer doesn't mean I'm not a mother, grandmother, friend, student, lover of books, music, the theater, and, incidentally, a *fisherwoman*. It does mean that I cannot ignore the reality of cancer in my life. Your awareness of my need for privacy is also a gift. Don't interpret it as a rejection of your efforts. I still need you to be sensitive in offering your support. Nevertheless, keep in mind that sometimes the line between being supportive and being intrusive is a fine one.

6 BE PATIENT WITH THE PATIENT TELLING IT LIKE IT IS

The most heartening news for anyone facing the threat of cancer today is that people can gain remission and even cures after treatment. But this does not diminish the realities of what the aftermath can bring. For those who have had major surgery, cancer means also seeing mastectomy scars, managing an ileostomy, or learning to speak through a mechanical device. Even if one had a very positive self-image before diagnosis, it takes a great deal of strength and faith to believe that in time complete health will be restored. In some cases, the cost will be great: sterility, impotence, temporary or permanent loss of libido, chemically induced diabetes, heart problems, premature cataracts, neuropathy (numbness of the fingers and toes), loss of muscle tone, even bone degeneration. In some cases, patients choose to go far from home to centers specializing in their cancer. Think about having some of these experiences 1,500 miles from friends and family. The true miracle is that most patients manage to rise to immense emotional and physical challenges.

Friends and family want us to be well. In that desire they may close their eyes to cancer realities like fear, pain, debilitation, anger, depression, and frustration that patients face daily. If you ignore those realities, you are really rejecting who the patient is during cancer time. Being patient with patients means trying to follow their timetable, not yours. Someone you care about is in cancer land. Neither you nor he wants him to be there. Expect good and bad moments, good and bad days, good and bad attempts at communication.

Cancer is now much more manageable than it was even a few years ago. Be patient with the patient. Please see him as he is, not as you want him to be. I don't want to have to perform as a patient. I don't want to have to deny that I'm feeling miserable just to protect you. I need to know that if I'm hurting, emotionally or physically, I can let it all out. I'm not obligated to cheer you up. I need to know you'll hear what I'm saying, even if it's painful. I may need to say I'm afraid I'm going to die. You do not want to hear it. Don't simply say everything will be all right. You're negating my fear. Wanting things to go right doesn't mean they will go right. No one knows. Just be there. When my mood darkens, accept that. Your words may help when my mood lightens, but don't censor my pain. Why is it that we can understand the physical pain of cancer, but often turn away from its emotional pain?

Does this mean you can never say what you think to the patient? Of course not. However, there is a need to acknowledge the yin and yang, the delicate balance of behavior. There is a time to speak, and a time to be silent, a time to suggest, and a time to listen. After diagnosis, during treatment and survival, the patient is not only undergoing major physical challenges, he is grieving as well. Careers may have to be put on hold. With many, pregnancy is no longer an option. Young men are routinely told to go to the sperm bank before they start chemotherapy or radiation. Dreams need to be postponed or changed. For those with young children, the question may be, "Will I see them graduate or marry?" For those of us who are older, it may be "Will my grandchildren remember me?" "Do I need to take early retirement?" "How will we pay for the services not covered by insurance?" Help the patient to accept the reality that sometimes a cancer diagnosis means things will never quite be the same again. There's LBC— life before cancer—and LAC—life after cancer, a new life calendar. Facing these mega-questions is almost insurmountable. Your presence, your acceptance, your patience, your love are what is needed.

Time has enormous impact on the patient. It's not waiting for the test result just for the initial diagnosis; it's waiting for the test results every time a cancer checkup is needed. The tests may be weekly, monthly, every three months. Instead of PMS (premenstrual syndrome), it's PMC (pre-medical checkup). When that cancer clock starts, friends and family need to recognize the start of a period of high anxiety. Even though it's been more than ten years since my diagnosis of multiple myeloma, the wait for the consultation is excruciating. Every cough for a lung cancer patient is frightening. Every backache can spell trouble for a myeloma patient. The swelling of a gland can be overwhelming for someone with lymphoma. One's life is literally under the microscope. During this waiting period the real life must again be put on hold. But which is the real life? Is it the cancer life or the non-cancer life? In truth, they both are.

Be patient with the patient as he or she tries to gain control during treatment. Ask, ask, ask. Don't assume you know what is needed. If you ask me what I need, I get a sense that I have some control. In your desire to help, don't take over. That can be counterproductive. If you let me do nothing, the message may be that I can do nothing. I need to feel competent. I need to feel that I am not a victim. Help me to do what I can.

During recovery, I was often told that I was doing too much. Perhaps I was. Trust the patient. Even today, my body tells me when to stop. True, there are times I fight the fatigue, but the patient needs to assert life even as she recognizes limitations. Selma Schimmel's book, *Cancer Talk,* recounts one patient speaking of her fatigue. She said, "Getting off the couch and going to bed is the highlight of my evening." At other times, the patient will force herself to perform routine household chores. Even taking out the garbage can be an affirming act.

Something very minor can trigger a negative reaction in a patient. Imagine the young woman who, in straightening up the medicine cabinet, finds a box of tampons. Her chemotherapy is over, but she hasn't had a period in months. She may be sterile. The tampon is another reminder of a loss. We expect the big things to have an impact on the patient—the drugs, the pain, the wig. Do not underestimate the impact of little things. I remember how traumatic it was for me to take all my bras and put them in the bag with other clothing I was planning to donate.

Ken Wilber's *Grace and Grit* is the story of Ken and Treya. A month before their wedding, Treya found a lump, a lump which was not the cyst everyone expected, but cancer. Theirs was a difficult struggle. At one point, they bought a Jeep Wrangler with a six-year warranty. Treyla wondered whether she would be around for the end of the warranty. Her thought was an entirely natural one. If your friend makes a similar kind of comment, listen and accept it. The pat response, "Of course you'll be around," won't work. If the patient were that confident, she wouldn't have made the statement. A better response might be, "When the warranty is up, I'll take you out for dinner."

When I was hospitalized, I had lipstick on my night table at all times. Except for one or two really bad days, I always managed to put lipstick on. It was my way of showing I still had some power over my situation. Anything you can do that demonstrates strength for the patient is good. It may be in encouraging your mother to get dressed, to get out of her hospital gown. It may be in offering to walk with your father around the hospital corridor, even if that means he has to drag an IV pole. It does not mean giving orders.

Surprisingly enough, you will also have to be patient when treatment ends. You would think that this time would be a cause for celebration, and it certainly is. Nevertheless, during chemotherapy, radiation, or physical therapy, patients are in a hospital environment or at least are seeing professionals on a routine basis. The medical calendar provides structure. Cancer life has a schedule. Patients are tended to, watched, their blood and vital signs monitored. There is medical safety.

When treatment ends, there is a void; the medical world has shrunk, and with it a certain security. Security must be built in new ways. It is here that friends and family can be most helpful, by creating new pathways of behavior to the world where the person can again be whole. For some patients, this period is what I call cancer withdrawal. Their medical family, for the most part, has gone. No one is tending to their every medical need. They're on your own. However, their feeling of medical isolation will soon pass. They will be medically emancipated.

KEEP YOUR EYES OPEN

The amount of medication some cancer patients take is overwhelming. One drug stops nausea, another prevents shingles. There are anti-fungal drugs and antibiotics. The list goes on. I still find it difficult to swallow large pills; I took so much medication for so long. Be aware of the impact of medications. There may be psychological as well as physical side effects. For example, steroids, often used in cancer treatment, can have significant, often negative effects on personality. Some patients on high doses of steroids are advised to hide their charge cards, since spree spending is a possibility. Insomnia can occur. Pain medications affect behavior. During the years I was on Interferon, I had flu-like symptoms constantly. The term "chemo brain," the inability to concentrate, is all too real for some of us. That loss of concentration is frightening.

If you think the patient is overreacting to a medication, or overreacting in general, you may want to ask how she's feeling at that moment. If the patient speaks of her inability to focus or stay on task, don't make light of it. If a condition merits her speaking about it, then that is important. There's nothing worse than broaching an issue and being told, "It's nothing." It may well be nothing. I don't like to complain, but if I do, please don't "pooh-pooh" it.

For some, not just the patient, being open and communicative comes naturally. For others, it can be like learning to drive a shift car. No one shifts smoothly the first time. When do I put my foot on the clutch, when on the brake, when on the gas pedal? The grinding of gears is painful to hear. Yet, suddenly, at some point, the mechanics become fixed in the driver's mind, and he can shift smoothly and effortlessly. Learning to be open will be the same for some patients and their friends and family. The first words will be difficult to say. Saying, "I have cancer" for the first time was painful for me. Accept the silences, the pauses, the verbal fragments. Ultimately, the verbal gears will mesh; communication will be established.

Recovery takes time. Sometimes only partial recovery occurs. There may be permanent effects from the treatment. No matter how much you want your friend or loved one to recover, it may be months before things seem normal again. No one wants to recover more than the patient does, but you can't mandate recovery. There are times when it will be difficult for the patient to go forward, to be positive. Acknowledge that pause in the process. It isn't your job to try to jolt the patient out of her listlessness or his temporary depression. It *is* your job to recognize the lull, accept, and watch it. If the pause, the depression, or the anxiety seems to linger, then you may try to talk about it, mention it to a family member or, if you're an immediate family member, to the doctor. Pushing gently at times may be good; dragging the patient forward beyond his limits isn't fair. Again, the delicate balance, the yin and yang.

During treatment, doctors, nurses, technicians are all giving instructions. What is needed is not more instructions from you, but a consistent acknowledgment that you're there. Let the patient make requests of you. Your being there, however, doesn't mean that the person with cancer has the right to say or do anything he chooses. The patient has leeway, not license.

The most important thing I ever wanted as a patient was to know that I wasn't alone. The cancer journey is a lonely one, even when we're surrounded by loved ones. We, too, have problems with what to say and what to do. We, too, fear showing our scars, be they real or emotional. We, too, feel guilt, if not over the disease, then over the pain we have caused those we know or love. Cancer attacks not only cells, but everything and everyone that is meaningful to us. No one is untouched. If I'm on cancer overload, I don't want to put you there as well.

In terms of overload, just think of a computer. There are two programs running simultaneously—the cancer program and the life program. During diagnosis and treatment, the cancer program is running in the foreground. During survivorship, the cancer program is running in the background. There is no denying the existence of both programs. You don't want the cancer program to cause the other to crash. Remembering that the life program is the primary program sometimes takes work, work you can help with.

7 THE PROFESSIONALS

The Oath of Hippocrates urges doctors "First, do no harm." This has been interpreted as doing no harm in terms of patient treatment. Its meaning now needs to be expanded so that physicians' words and actions also do no harm. Those who choose a career in medicine must be as responsible for what they say and what they do as they are for their recommendations for medication and treatment. Indeed, so much attention is paid to what medical personnel say and do that their cancer etiquette, or lack of it, will sometimes have a greater impact on the patient than that of anyone else with whom he or she interacts.

Medical personnel see cancer patients all the time. They see pain, and a complete range of human emotions: fear, anger, confusion, depression, frustration, and anxiety, to mention just a few. They see patients whose entire lives have been turned upside down. Instead of career goals, social events, meetings, long-range plans, cancer takes front stage. All else fades into the background. Think of how overwhelmed we are in dealing with just one person going through the cancer experience. How do those who have chosen oncology as a specialty cope with dealing with cancer every minute of their working day, every year of their professional lives? It must be extraordinarily difficult and stressful. The truth is that some do better than others. Nevertheless, as professionals, they must be accountable for the impact of their behavior.

WHAT THEY'VE SAID

Previously, I've alluded to some of the objectionable comments made to patients often by well-meaning friends, family, colleagues, and loved ones. How have doctors, nurses, staff, technologists erred? Dominick

Dunne, the author, switched doctors when his physician had his nurse call him with the diagnosis of prostate cancer. It's difficult enough to get a cancer diagnosis on the phone; there is no doctor so esteemed that he can't deal directly with his patient at this most critical moment.

One breast cancer patient heard her cancer diagnosis over the phone on a Friday afternoon. After talking to her, the doctor said, "Have a good weekend." This knee-jerk comment is unacceptable at a time like that. Yes, maybe he had to tell three other patients of their diagnoses, but he still must remember that every patient is an individual, not a tumor. Saying, "This is a bad way to start a weekend, but you and your family will now have an opportunity to talk over your options. I'll call you next week," would have been infinitely better.

In another instance, Steve M., a myeloma patient, went for a routine visit to his ophthalmologist. Making casual conversation, the doctor said to him, "Isn't that regarded as a death sentence?" The statement would have been inappropriate even from a lay person. From a physician, it was horribly chilling.

A radiologist, in speaking to a patient with a mass, called a plasmacytoma, said, "If you don't get chemo, you'll die." This statement may have been true. However, there is telling the truth, and there is telling the truth. Saying, "Chemotherapy is an absolute necessity in your case. Without it, you will greatly decrease your chances for recovery," is also the truth, but the effect of those words will be less devastating.

An oncology patient queried her doctor about her cholesterol level. He answered, "Don't worry about your cholesterol. Your death certificate will say ovarian cancer." Yes, ovarian cancer is often fatal. One consistent goal of cancer etiquette is to remember that the cancer patient is still an individual, someone with a career, family, interests, hopes, and dreams. The medical staff, too, must keep that in mind. How much better it would have been had he said, "Your cholesterol is too high. You've been through so much with the ovarian cancer, we're not going to let your cholesterol get out of control."

A friend of mine, accompanied by his wife, went to his urologist's office to discuss the results of his biopsy. After keeping them waiting for an hour, which seemed like an eternity, the urologist opened the door, poked his head in, and announced in a cold-as-ice manner, "You're a very sick man. You have cancer, and your kidney has to be removed. You'll have to excuse me—I'm in a very important golf tournament, and I'm already late for it. Talk to you tomorrow." And with an airy wave, he disappeared!

My friends were shocked speechless. Then shock turned to anger at the offhand delivery of such disastrous news, with no opportunity for them to acquire more information. Needless to say, they sought medical care elsewhere. The kidney was subsequently removed, and my friend resumed his normal life.

The author, Louise Albert, visited her gynecologist for a checkup. When he finished, Louise asked him if he would please do a breast examination as well. He said, "What for? You do them, don't you?" She responded, "I would still feel better if you did it." A breast exam is usually a routine part of a gynecological exam. He did the exam reluctantly, and actually did discover a lump in one of her breasts. He then joked, "Well, that's what you get when you ask for a breast exam!" To add insult to injury, he suggested a general surgeon for Louise to use. She asked, "Wouldn't it be better if a breast surgeon did it?" He looked at her, threw up his arms, and in an annoyed, impatient tone spurted, "Oh, I don't have time for this." Louise did not have time for him either. She never saw him again.

Vivian's experience was equally disturbing. She had gone for a consultation regarding a possible breast cancer diagnosis. She knew she had picked the wrong doctor when he said, "Don't worry. We'll save your 'boobies.' " She took offense, right or wrong, at his lack of professionalism in using the vernacular, "boobies." This was a critical medical moment for her, and she felt his condescending attitude was inappropriate.

A physician, whose mother was being treated for cancer, might expect but not necessarily receive special attention for her. Linda Villarosa, in an article in *The New York Times*, writes of Dr. Larry A. Green, who participated in a study evaluating the care of such patients. His interest in the topic had been spurred by his dissatisfaction with the treatment his mother, a stomach cancer patient, received. He found errors of judgment, and lack of attention to her needs. The low point occurred weeks after she had had her stomach removed. She was still in the hospital. Dr. Green found her sitting in a wheelchair, vomiting into a pan. Her doctor entered the room, and his first comment to her was, "Mrs. Green, I told you it would be difficult to get along without a stomach." Where was the greeting? Where was the compassion? He might have said, "I'm sorry you've had such a difficult time since your surgery." He didn't even say, "I'll examine you and see if there's anything else I can do to make you more comfortable."

There needs to be dignity in every interaction between physician and patient. For example, doctors occasionally check on patients during their chemotherapy session. The treatment area can be large, with many patients receiving treatment simultaneously. Recliners are close together. Patients, friends and family often talk about their status with their chemo neighbors. Physicians must be particularly careful in this or any other public setting not to discuss issues of prognosis or metastasis, lest other patients overhear those private conversations.

POSSIBILITIES

As I suggested earlier, even changing one word may change a statement from an unacceptable one to an acceptable one. Natalie Davis Spingarn in *The New Cancer Survivors* tells of a woman whose husband was diagnosed with pancreatic cancer, a cancer very difficult to treat and usually fatal. The resident physician asked him, "What was your profession?" His wife complained and suggested that the question should have been what *is* his profession. The doctor called her an optimist. Clearly, the diagnosis was a terrible one. If a patient's days are numbered, the doctor must at least give him the opportunity of living those days to the best of his ability, with his professional identity intact. Setting a doomsday date, or denying all hope is unacceptable. Better to say, "The chances for long-term survival are not good. We'll do all we can. We need to be realistic, but we don't need to deny hope." More words may be needed, but those might be just the ones that enable the patient to go on in spite of the devastation of the diagnosis. Dr. Jerome Groopman writes that more than thirty times a month an oncologist has to give a cancer diagnosis, tell a patient of a recurrence, indicate that a treatment is no longer working. That can never be easy. Doctors know that medicine is powerful. Words concerning cancer are equally powerful. There should be a sacred consideration to those a doctor uses.

Even the professionals providing support services must mind their words. A nutritionist in speaking to a patient said, "I don't know why you have lung cancer; you eat the right things." The nutritionist meant to compliment the patient; yet her words failed. "The fact that you've followed a good diet all along will make it easier for you to continue good nutrition as you recover" would have been a better choice of words.

Ruth G. battled cancer for many years. She refused to give up, enduring extensive chemotherapy. During the last four months of her life, except during the periods when she was hospitalized, the same physical therapist came to her home three times a week. She got to know Ruth and the family. When Ruth died, her husband was surprised that the physical therapist neither called nor sent a card. This is a delicate area. When should medical personnel extend condolences? Do they need to have known the patient one month, two months, three months? What are the parameters? Should they at least call the family? Should the agency that sends nurses and physical therapists set guidelines for this circumstance? There are no rules here. My gut reaction is that if a doctor, nurse, or therapist has had a very long relationship with a patient, some recognition of that relationship is appropriate. The issue merits discussion among the professionals.

The truth is that those in the medical community need to think before they speak, just as the rest of us have to. The bad news is that too many of them are unaware—or worse, indifferent—to the power of their words. The good news is that many, many physicians, nurses, receptionists, and technicians are caring and thoughtful.

The issue of how well or how poorly physicians communicate with their patients is not a new one. In 1926, Dr. Francis Weld Peabody addressed students at the Harvard Medical School. Much of what he said then is still true today. He spoke of how young graduates know about the "mechanism of disease, but very little about the practice of medicine." He went on to say, "The treatment of a disease may be entirely impersonal; the care of a patient must be completely personal." The patient has the right to expect to be treated as an individual, not a number, a kidney, or a lung. The doctor who sees only the tumor and not the whole person may have sound medical skills but does not know the art of medicine. If the patient is willing to accept this one-dimensional approach to treatment, that is his option. However, patients have a right to expect more; the physician has the responsibility to provide more.

Ironically, the advances in medical technology may contribute to the distance between medical professionals and patients. Does technology limit humanism? Even the language of medicine, increasingly technical, makes it more difficult to communicate. Some physicians seem to hide behind the jargon rather than to take the time to translate "medicalese" to understandable English. Dr. Peabody would probably have a lot to say about that today.

Catherine, a physician, cried when she learned of her diagnosis. A colleague quickly gave her a prescription for Valium. Catherine suggested that crying was the right thing to do under the circumstances. She remained open about her situation, worked during treatment, and volunteered to speak to three groups of interns about her illness. Dr. Barron Lerner wrote, "Many at the session, accustomed to hiding their emotions, wept openly." Still, on at least two occasions, she received less than caring treatment from her colleagues. Lerner said that one doctor, in front of Catherine, loudly criticized another doctor on the treatment choice. Another physician did not return her calls. How can a doctor not return a call from another doctor? She wouldn't have called unless there was a sound medical reason. Her suggestions for her peers were that they be "frank, attentive and patient." She encouraged emotional connection, rather than distance from the patient. Dr. Peabody would have been proud of her.

Dr. Kathleen Ogle wrote of a patient, a former dean of students, who was dying. The patient asked for a pass to see a local theater production of *The Gospel at Colonus*, based on the Oedipus story. The medical staff refused the pass, concerned that she could catch an infection. Dr. Ogle was at the performance, and realized how much it would have meant to the patient. Ironically, the woman died a short time later, of an infection she picked up at the hospital. Ogle says that setting priorities not be reserved for the physician only. The patient has the right to participate. Dr. Ogle suggests that the white coat can blind the doctor. She says, "Perhaps that is why we looked at a patient ravaged by cancer and recited a litany of facts . . . but failed to see her humanity. Oedipus plucked out his eyes; do physicians strap on their own blinders?"

THE CHALLENGE

There is a challenge in treating a cancer patient. The individual who is difficult to get along with before cancer will probably be just as difficult after diagnosis. The couple whose marriage is troubled is certainly not likely to have marital strains relieved after the diagnosis. Cancer can intensify who we are, but doesn't *change* who we are, at least not at first. Thus, the oncology staff has to deal with not just the "good" patient, however that is defined, but with all patients. There are those who are disturbed emotionally, those who have multiple physical problems, those who are under enormous financial strain, those who may be totally alone, those whose native language is not English, those whose home life is troubled. The surprise is not that some doctors and nurses are curt, uncommunicative and officious, but that so many treat us with skill, tenderness, and great humanity.

A survey for the Association of American Medical Colleges found that 85 percent of patients chose their physicians on the basis of the doctor's communication skills. In addition, 77 percent cited how important it was that the physician be able to explain complicated medical procedures. Admittedly, doctors are pressured. They have too many patients, too many forms to fill out, too many new techniques and protocols to learn. These are not good enough excuses. Poor communication can be so detrimental to the patient's recovery that it cannot be ignored.

What is being done to improve the communication, the connection between the medical staff and the patient? What works? What doesn't? Certainly the time spent with the patient is a primary component. If the doctor appears to have no time for the patient, the patient can only react negatively, either verbally, or emotionally. In *The New Cancer Survivors,* by Natalie Spingarn, Dr. Tom Fahey stresses that patients need to believe the doctor has time for the patient. "To stand by the doorstop or at the entrance to the patient's room and look like you're ready to fly down the hall is just terribly disturbing to people."

IT DOESN'T TAKE MUCH

Evan Handler was often dissatisfied with the behavior of his physicians. At one point, a new doctor asked permission to come into his room. Handler says, "I found his demeanor to be exquisitely sensitive to the fact that he had come into the temporary home of another individual." Doctors need to do whatever they can to preserve the patient's sense of self, of individuality. Robert Lipsyte is absolutely right when, *In the Country of Illness*, he says, "We don't need socialized medicine as badly as we need more socialized people practicing medicine."

These suggestions—asking permission to enter a room, looking the patient in the eye, letting the patient feel that he is the center of the doctor's attention—need no legislation. These actions will not increase the cost of medical care. How much time would it really take if a doctor sat down rather than stood as he spoke to the patient? Those few extra moments might mean fewer calls later on, because patients had the time to ask the questions they needed to ask. Furthermore, doctors who delay in returning calls for days simply cause more anxiety in the patient. This anxiety is likely to produce even more calls.

The patient-doctor relationship is obviously not an equal one. Now, with more and more patients seeking and getting information about their disease, there has been somewhat of a shift. But no one would ever consider the relationship to be equal. Therefore, physicians must do whatever they can to make the patient feel that there is some parity, even though it cannot be medical parity. In its simplest form, the doctor must remember that the patient's life has as much value as the surgeon's. Dr. Kate O'Hanlan, an oncological gynecologist at the Stanford University Medical Center, has the right attitude. She says, "I want patients to feel I'm their healer, not their plumber."

Years ago, the physician would recommend a treatment and the patient, in all likelihood, would have accepted the recommendation. Today that model is less common. Dr. Peter A. Ubel writes of a patient who had been diagnosed with prostate cancer. A urologist had recommended removal of the prostate. The patient's wife wanted him to investigate radiation possibilities. A friend of the patient had avoided both alternatives by choosing a "watch and wait" option. So, in addition to medical criteria, the patient's values must be part of the treatment equation. As Dr. Ubel comments, ". . . a man who cares little about the risk of impotence is better suited to surgical treatment of his prostate cancer than a man who highly values sexual function." Some patients want to be part of the decision-making process. Others, however, still prefer to defer to the doctor. Physicians can learn from Dr. Ubel's perceptions: "I've learned that the distinction between letting patients make decisions and making decisions for them is often very subtle."

THE ETIQUETTE OF TIME

It is my body; my decisions ultimately will help to decide my fate. It will take time for the doctor to help me arrive at what may be the best decision. This is time the physician must give. Ultimately, if the patient and doctor work as a team, time will be saved; at the very least, there may be less fear for the patient.

There is an etiquette of time even with regard to tests. Yes, the radiology staff have films to read, the pathologists have slides to examine, the phlebotomists have vials of blood to evaluate. Yet, if a member of the cleri-cal staff could call the patient and say approximately when they will process the test results, that will make the patient feel that there is concern and interest on the part of the doctor or the lab. At the very least, every ef-fort should be made to get test results to a patient before the start of a weekend. There is nothing worse than waiting over a weekend to learn whether or not a biopsy is positive. A few extra moments do mean a lot.

Time is particularly important when the patient, accompanied by his or her spouse, significant other, or family member, consults with the on-cologist. At times, I've waited for two hours to see Dr. Jagannath, my myeloma oncologist, but once I enter his examining room, time stops. Even during routine checkups, he speaks slowly, answers all my ques-tions, and draws diagrams if necessary. At those times, I am his only pa-tient. He has never made a call while he's meeting with me, unless it is an emergency or to consult regarding my condition. That's good medicine.

When Alice Trillin consulted her doctor as to whether her lung cancer had reoccurred, the doctor said, ". . . I will tell you what we can do. I will also tell you what I think you should do, and then you can make up your mind." How wonderful; the doctor was not only encouraging the patient's participation in the decision-making process, he was acknowledging that it is, in the end, the patient's decision to make. That's medical etiquette.

Adding to the difficulty in communication about cancer is the fact that doctors are obligated to tell patients the truth. If the patient and family don't know the reality of the situation, they cannot make informed deci-sions regarding treatment. How to tell the truth is the doctor's challenge; how to hear the truth is the patient's. Dr. Richard Stock, who treated Mayor Rudolph Guiliani for prostate cancer, said he would never tell a pa-tient he had six months to live. "There's always that small percentage of patients that defies the odds, and if I can give a patient the hope that maybe they're in that percentage, well, I know that's what I would want if it was me in their shoes."

Surgeons save lives, but they don't often have the opportunity to de-velop substantive relations with their patients. Once the patient leaves the hospital, he usually doesn't see the surgeon until it is time for the stitches to come out, drains to be removed, or a physical exam. Wouldn't it be great if the surgeon could take a minute or two to call after the patient ar-rives at home? A follow-up call is often made by the hospital to a patient who's had ambulatory surgery. Why can't the surgeon call the patient after major cancer surgery? It's the right thing to do, and it would mean a lot. How many calls a day would that be?

In contrast, Lance Armstrong writes in *It's Not About the Bike: My Journey Back to Life*, about his special relationship with his oncology nurse, LaTrice Haney. After an important checkup, it was the doctor who suggested Haney call Lance with the good results. Here the nurse's call was not because the doctor was too busy. It was that the doctor knew Lance would be happy to hear the news from his exceptional nurse.

NURSES ARE SPECIAL

Doctors often ask nurses to do what they may not want to, such as giving bad news or dealing with uncomfortable family situations. In spite of the pressure that nurses work under, they act professionally, gallantly, and with amazing kindness and grace. Their etiquette batting average is high. They somehow instinctively know how to act. They deserve our respect and attention. Yet, they too are human, and like all of us will have moments of curtness, aloofness, or impatience. Even nurses don't do it right all the time. Nurses often have the additional task of being the buffer between the patient and the doctor. If the nurse has a good relationship with the doctor, he or she can strengthen connection between the physician and the patient. She becomes the linchpin in the relationship.

One nurse wrote that working with cancer patients reminds her of the preciousness of life. Cheryl believes she became a better nurse when she gave up trying to say the perfect thing to the patient or his family. She also found that at times silence is often the best way to communicate. Tears and hugs also work well for her. When one of her favorite patients, a 22-year-old leukemia patient, relapsed, all Cheryl could do was hug her patient and say she loved her. Is this unprofessional? Perhaps it may seem so to some, but not to me, and certainly not to the young woman she comforted.

Years ago, patients stayed in the hospital for weeks. Now a woman is often released a day or so after she's had a mastectomy, a man two or three days after prostate surgery. This doesn't allow much time to build relationships. Somehow, nurses manage to succeed even in a short time. Sometimes, though, even nurses need to step back. Sometimes, it is that a patient has touched her in a particular way. Sometimes, it is that the patient is particularly demanding. Sometimes, it is that the patient reminds her of something painful in her own life. What's important is that nurses realize they can't be perfect all the time. When those moments occur, a nurse will sometimes ask her colleague to take care of the patient at that particular time, or for that particular shift. Nurses admit they're human.

LITTLE THINGS

Hospital staffs are beginning more and more to understand that little things do mean a lot to cancer patients. Patients who travel to large cancer centers often must be away for weeks or even months at a time. One patient, Bob M., was receiving treatment at the Fred Hutchinson Cancer Research Center in Seattle. His wife tells of a Christmas party the hospital gave for their transplant patients. The staff served refreshments. There were games so that patients could get acquainted. Patients had their pictures taken with Santa Claus. There were tables with gifts on them. The sign on the table said, "You can't go out to the stores, so we brought the stores to you." At the end of the celebration, patients were given baskets filled with treats, phone calling cards, shampoo, toys, etc.

Johns Hopkins Hospital in Baltimore has an evening of elegance the night before the transplant patient goes home. A waiter in a tuxedo serves the patient and his guest wine and the patient's choice of food. Fran was in the transplant unit at the University of Connecticut, where she felt like a "pampered guest." Those who brought her meals did not wear uniforms. Their clothing included a maroon vest, white shirt, and bow tie. Cloth mats and napkins added a sense of class. The hospital's efforts made her feel that her stay was "less sterile, more comforting, and much more bearable. That feeling of having a bright red C on my chest just wasn't there."

Obviously, these forms of celebration are not financially feasible for every institution. Still, the medical community can develop symbolic ways to acknowledge the special situation that cancer patients face. Like many medical centers, every spring, White Plains Hospital participates in National Cancer Survivors Day. They invite all cancer survivors and their families for a spectacular outdoor brunch. A speaker acknowledges the special day, and everyone has a wonderful time.

Years ago, I decided to have a party for longtime employees. Every time someone left the library for another job or to retire, we had had a party. I decided we needed a party to honor those who stayed. Every staff member who had worked at the library for more than five years was given a large felt S. Those who worked in the library fewer than five years received a smaller S. I wrote an individualized letter of congratulations to everyone, for the special work he or she was doing. Some cancer patients get a token present or diploma as they leave the hospital. We graduate from school; why can't we graduate from chemotherapy or radiation?

At my local hospital, the nurses are sensitive to the transition that occurs when a patient finishes chemotherapy. One woman had weekly treatments for nearly a year. From where she sat, she could see a picture hanging on the wall outside of her room. She felt that picture helped her deal with the treatments. On the last day of treatment, she saw someone take the picture down from the wall. "What are they doing with my picture?" she asked. Actually, the picture was being taken down so that the oncology nurses could give it to her as their gift. For that patient, it was the perfect choice.

EVEN DOCTORS CAN LEARN

The medical profession is becoming more and more aware of the importance of connection and communication. It may be too late to train the doctors who have always been short with patients, always in a hurry, often lacking in humanity, but changes are occurring. John Langone, writing in *The New York Times*, reports that at Yale University, newly enrolled medical students are given their white coats, their "cloaks of compassion," and they recite a "Human Relations Code of Conduct." Today, more than 70 medical schools in the United States offer courses in spirituality, or include spirituality as part of the curriculum. At the Medical University of South Carolina College of Medicine, students attend seminars dealing with faith, tragedy, the limits of healing, and related topics. At Harvard, first-year medical students visit patients who have life-threatening illnesses. They are expected to build relationships with the patients and their families. Also at Harvard, in one elective course, if a student has a patient who dies, the student is encouraged to attend the wake, the funeral, and to share in the family's grief. In 1998, the first Chair of Palliative Medicine in the United States was created at the Albert Einstein College of Medicine. The acknowledgment that pain treatment is a critical part of care is an important step. This list of positive changes should grow in future years.

Dr. Peabody would welcome these changes. When he spoke at Harvard those many years ago, he knew he had cancer. He could identify when he said that the clinical picture of a patient is "not just a photograph of a man sick in bed; it is an impressionistic painting of the patient surrounded by his home, his work, his relations, his friends, his joys, sorrows, hopes and fears." He could well have been talking about himself.

The torch has passed from Dr. Peabody to Dr. Jerome Groopman. Like Peabody, Groopman is a professor at Harvard Medical School. He, too, understands that knowing the patient as an individual is critical. Medical technique, research, technology, surgery, chemistry are important, but they are not enough. Dr. Groopman, in *The Anatomy of Hope*, writes that "true hope has proved as important as any medication I might prescribe or any procedure I might perform." He knows that although hope may be intangible, it should not be ignored or demeaned as a factor in the patient's care. He knows that physicians must expand their medical lens so that they see beyond the physical.

Dr. Bernie Siegel, in *How to Live Between Office Visits,* stresses how important listening is as a tool. "When someone you love has difficulties, listen. When you're feeling terrible that you can't provide a cure, listen. When you don't know what to offer the people you care about, listen, listen, listen."

Friends, patients, and caregivers would do well to heed the words of these wise physicians. They need to apply those words as they relate to the doctors, nurses, and staff they meet. Saying to a member of the medical staff, "You don't know how I feel" might or might not be true. Doctors, nurses, receptionists, and technicians find cancer in their lives as well. However, they have to leave their personal stories at the door when they enter the office or hospital, so that they can focus on each patient. If we expect the doctors to look upon us as complex individuals, we must do the same with and for them.

Sometimes, it is a personal issue that causes a physician to change his attitude toward his patients. Dr. Rachel Naomi Remem was treating a cancer surgeon for depression. The surgeon said, "I knew cancer very well, but I did not know people before." She tells of another surgeon whose wife was diagnosed with cancer. The surgeon decided to make origami cranes, 1,000 of them, in an effort to help his wife heal. He gave the cranes to his patients, one of whom said, "And he made it for me. How could I possibly not heal?" Remembering that we're dealing with an individual who happens to have cancer changes the equation.

As patients, friends, and family, we all have etiquette responsibilities to the doctor and others in the medical community. We're in a relationship. They, in turn, have a responsibility to us. We should not expect the doctor to be the major emotional support of the patient. That is our job. The doctor can recommend and encourage counseling and support groups, but it is unfair to expect him or her to deal with the myriad emotional issues that are linked to cancer. Doctors must be sensitive to the issues, but their primary focus must be on treating the patient.

We also need to be careful not to direct our anger and frustrations about the cancer to the medical staff. Yes, the insurance company has been denying claims. Yes, the doctor has kept me waiting in the waiting room for over an hour. Yes, they said the medical records would be ready, but the fax still has not been sent to the consultant. These are real concerns, but let's assign blame when appropriate. If it's the medical staff, tell them. If a doctor is continuously curt and inattentive, one has the prerogative to change doctors. We need to remind ourselves that the doctors and nurses are not responsible for the cancer; they are responsible for treating the cancer. They really are trying to do their best. We'll have to deal with our personal frustrations in other venues.

People with cancer often try to transform themselves into medical Olympians—not so easy. They want to reach the finish line, the end of treatment as soon as possible. They will falter; they may want to quit the race, yet most struggle on. If excellence is needed to succeed, then excellence must be demanded of everyone. Those specializing in oncology can serve as models for the rest of us. If we see them relating to patients, if we see them taking the time to communicate with the patients, if we see them listening to what the patients have to say, then the rest of us can model our behavior on theirs.

IT'S OK TO LAUGH

Did you laugh today? Probably. Was it a joke, an e-mail message, a comment made by someone at work, a television show, a pun, or a new word spoken by your toddler? Often we forget what stimulated the laugh, but no one denies its value. We know that laughter nourishes us. Norman Cousins, in *Anatomy of an Illness*, describes how laughter proved to be the best medicine in his struggle for health. In *A Little Book of Nurses' Rules,* Hammerschmidt and Meador comment that laughter is "free, nonfattening, salt free, without side effects, and available for use by anyone. Best of all, it is contagious."

Even in the midst of tragedy, humor surfaces. Former Mayor Rudolph Giuliani knows the power of laughter. At a Carnegie Hall Benefit, a month after the World Trade Center bombing, he said to the audience, "I'm here to give you permission to laugh. And if you don't, I'll have you arrested." If humor is so terrific, how can there be caveats when it comes to humor and cancer?

Earlier, I spoke of how upset I was when I told a friend about my breast cancer diagnosis and the need for a double mastectomy. Her response was that at least I would be symmetrical. I was speaking with her perhaps an hour or so after I had learned the biopsy results. Her joke at that moment was inappropriate. Had she made the same comment weeks later, my reaction would probably have been different. Verbal shock does not excuse verbal excess, even in the name of humor. Timing is everything.

Less than 48 hours after my breast surgery, I was talking on the phone with my daughter. When Jean asked how I was feeling, rather than saying that the catheter had been removed, I said, "I'm tubeless and boobless." Not such a great joke, but it seemed funny to both of us. Why was my remark acceptable yet my friend's was not? The difference is that the humor came from me. This is important to remember. When the patient is ready to laugh, be there to join in. That time may vary from patient to patient. It may depend on whether or not there has been surgery, and how serious the surgery was. It may depend on the stage of the cancer. It may depend on your relationship to the patient. It may depend on the patient's physical reactions to radiation or chemotherapy. It may even depend on the age of the patient. Even if you get a laugh one day, or the patient says something humorous, the humor valve may be turned off the next. My suggestion is to hold the jokes for a while, at least at the beginning, but be prepared to laugh. You never know when the patient will be ready to turn to humor as a healing mechanism.

Somehow, in spite of the diagnosis, the pain, the depression, the side effects of drugs, humor surfaces. In life, we often use black humor to get us through difficult times. Having cancer is certainly such a time. Humor, at least temporarily, holds back the cancer. Author Robert Lipsyte speaks of "tumor humor." He, too, emphasizes that the humor must come first from the patient. He considers humor coming from those "who haven't the right to use it" as offensive. Clearly, one should not make light of what the patient is going through. When the patient is ready to laugh about his or her situation, you'll hear about it. Then you can join in.

PATIENTS' HUMOR

Some of the following examples may seem sophomoric; others may not seem to be funny at all. Perhaps the bar for cancer humor needs to be set a bit lower. What's important is not that the patient came out with a brilliant bon mot, a clever pun, or a convoluted joke. What matters is that the patient found something to laugh about. There are so many moments of crying; any attempt at humor should be welcomed. Every laugh means one less tear.

For example, Anne is bald from chemotherapy. She and her friend Nina swim together at the local Y. When their pool closed for repairs, they had to go to another site. In the unfamiliar locker room after the swim, Nina asked Anne if she knew where the outlets for the hairdryers were. Her friend "dryly" replied, "I don't have to think about that." She was able to take her baldness and turn it into a moment for laughter.

In *Hope Lives* by Margit Esser Porter, a young woman recounts her adjustment to no longer getting her menstrual period. The periods had stopped because she had had a bone marrow transplant. What should she do with the super economy package of sanitary napkins that were in her closet? She stuck one on each foot, and skated around her hardwood floors clearing the dust. Instead of crying about her situation, she found a way to see the humor in it.

Another patient found that having cancer could be a real help when it came to telemarketers. He tells the caller he has cancer. There is silence, a "sorry to have bothered you" and a good bye. Who has the last laugh?

Recently, I had some back pain. I thought it was just a muscle strain, and called my daughter, Leslie, who is a physical therapist. She suggested an exercise: "Take your left elbow and move it over to your right boob." I interrupted and said, "If I had a right boob. . . ." She retorted, "C'mon Mom, cut me some slack," and we laughed. Nothing profound, nothing earthshakingly funny, but the fact that we can laugh about one of the most painful experiences in our lives is a good sign.

Margaret Edson uses sardonic humor in her play, *Wit*. The play's heroine, a professor of 17th-century poetry, is receiving high-dose chemotherapy as part of an experimental protocol. She resents the "how-are-you-feeling-today?" question. "I have been asked as I was emerging from a four-hour operation with a tube in every orifice, 'How are you feeling today?' I am waiting for the moment when someone asks me this question and I am dead." Edson's play reminds us that some oncologists see only numbers and are blind to the patient.

Since cancer affects how we feel about our sexuality, our body image, our attractiveness, our ability to laugh at ourselves under those circumstances is to be applauded. In spite of everything, we still look forward to and can joke about a social life after cancer. Gail C. suggests a dating service for cancer survivors. She talked about the idea with a male friend. His suggested name for such a group was "Fatal Attractions." Margit Esser Porter writes of one woman who, returning to dating after her mastectomy, saw new meaning in the term SWF, single white female.

Another woman, Bonnie T., has metastatic cancer. The oncologist told her that a recent bone survey had revealed a new lesion on her skull. Her comment was, "Well that's just what I need. Another hole in my head." Had the doctor said that to the patient, it would have been insensitive. Her ability to laugh at her own condition represents the best in cancer humor. Her self-deprecation gave her some control in an uncontrollable situation.

Catharine Honeyman knows when to laugh at herself. A large-breasted woman, she had been considering breast reduction. When an eight-centimeter breast tumor was found, she opted for a mastectomy. She called the insurance company many times, and fought with them until they finally approved a double mastectomy. In the operating room, just as the doctor was about to start the anesthesia, she gasped, "Doc, Doc! There's something I gotta get off my chest!" Since everyone in the O.R. knew how she felt about her breasts, they were all able to laugh at her "cutting" wit.

We know how security has affected air travel since September 11, 2001. I was flying from Ft. Lauderdale to Atlanta. When I went to check my bag at curbside, I was told they couldn't accept it. I went to the baggage check-in. There I was escorted to an alcove, where my bag was searched. The computer had picked me for a random search. The two women went over every piece in my bag. Was I upset or angry? No. My thought was that I was glad I was wearing my prostheses. Imagine if they'd searched and found two false "boobs" in the suitcase. To me, it seemed funny.

Lila Keary was tired of the trite phrases tossed at her. A friend said, "They tell me you're a little under the weather." Her response was, "You're kidding—they tell me I have cancer. Do you think there's been some kind of mix-up?"

Patients know people care about and for them. Nevertheless, at times the good intentions of those friends and family can be wearing. Humor can become a friendly weapon for patients at such times. Wendy's story appears in *The First Look* by Amelia Davis. Wendy discovered a lump on her breast just before her 23rd birthday. She sensed that some people felt she must have been responsible for the cancer. "Too much peanut butter" as a kid was her response to them. That seemed scientific enough for them.

Kathy used humor against an insensitive doctor. She had been using a handicapped parking permit for a serious knee problem. It was time for the permit to be renewed. She had had a double mastectomy and was still struggling with the effects of the chemotherapy, and added that as an explanation to the doctor. He said, "How do I know you had a double mastectomy?" One would think it's not something a woman would lie about. What did Kathy do? She just pulled up her shirt and showed her chest. She got the permit. Never underestimate a cancer patient.

A volunteer and cancer survivor, Emily Hollenberg, has a humor column online for the University of Michigan. She uses the David Letterman format of a list. Two of my favorites in her "Top 11 Ways to Know You Are a Cancer Survivor" are "When your biggest annual celebration is again your birthday, not the day you were diagnosed," and "When you use your Visa card more than your insurance card."

Dan Shapiro, author of *Mom's Marijuana*, was diagnosed at age 20 with Hodgkin's disease. The tumor was huge. He underwent years of treatment and is now in remission. Outstanding doctors, humor, and his mom's marijuana helped him along his path to recovery. Early on, just after his first radiation, Shapiro went to the local hardware store, purchased a spray can of lime green paint, and sprayed his chest to show what the radiation had done to him. His mother calmly looked at him and said, "I hope you didn't get paint on anything in your bedroom." Humor need not be one-sided.

Among the many items Shapiro brought to his hospital room was a huge water pistol. At one point, a team of doctors came to his room at a time when he was feeling particularly lousy. The lead doctor, a young man, started describing Dan's case. Dan asked who he was. There was no response. The resident continued with the litany of symptoms. Again, Shapiro asked who he was. No response. Shapiro asked him to stop talking. He didn't. What should he do? Shapiro drew out his trusty water gun, aimed, and shot it at the doctor. The resident and his retinue quickly left. Days later, the guilty resident asked permission to enter Dan's room, asked how he was feeling, discussed his case, prescribed medication, and left. The water treatment worked. They became friends. I don't recommend this solution for everyone, but it certainly was a creative approach. Dan's aim was true. The resident needed to be reminded that the patient had a persona, a personality, and a life, not merely a case number.

Cancer humor often occurs most easily when the patient talks to close friends or family. In her book, *Cancer Has Its Privileges*, Christine Clifford demonstrated her sense of humor, and she did so in front of thousands of people. Christine is a passionate golf fan. Between treatments, she and her husband decided to attend a professional tournament. She was standing behind the fairway ropes when a sudden gust of wind blew her hat and wig right into the middle of the fairway. There was a sudden silence; everyone looked at Christine. She calmly walked to the fairway, put her "hair" back where it belonged and calmly said, "Gentlemen, the wind is blowing from left to right." When it comes to gutsy cancer humor, Christine should get a trophy.

Beth Murphy writes in *Fighting for Our Future* about very young women who have breast cancer. Kathy Burgau is one of those women. She is also a jock. Her experience took place on a softball field, not a golf course. Kathy went back to playing softball two months after completing breast cancer chemotherapy. Sliding into base after blasting a triple, Kathy heard her friend say, "Kathy, adjust yourself." Momentarily confused, Kathy looked down and realized that her "boob" had fallen down to her stomach. She took out the offending prosthesis and threw it at her friend. Needless to say, when Kathy decided on reconstruction, she made sure to set the schedule so that the surgery would not conflict with the volleyball or softball seasons.

A few of my own memories come to mind. I was in the transplant center in Little Rock. It was late in the evening. My daughter, Jean, and I were in my hospital bed playing with a small hand-held poker game. We were competing with every deal, and laughing so hard that the nurses came in. They were surprised and delighted to hear laughter on a floor where so many were so ill. How could we laugh under those circumstances? Well, it certainly was better than crying. We were together. We were far from home. We loved each other. The game gave us permission to have fun. The nurses welcomed our humanity, our link to the non-cancer part of our world.

Before I started chemotherapy after my breast surgery, I was fitted with a new wig. Jean, her husband, Rick, and my daughter, Leslie, were visiting. Their children were asleep. I went into my room, put the wig on over my own hair, and we continued our conversation. After about a half-hour, I pulled my wig off and they roared. They hadn't even noticed. If my own children didn't recognize my wearing a wig, I knew things would be all right.

Last year, still not quite fully recuperated from my breast surgery and chemotherapy, I was in Atlanta helping to take care of my three grandchildren. My son-in-law's mother, Fran, and I were bathing our two granddaughters. They had frolicked quite a while when Fran said, "Time to pull the plug." "Fran," I said, "you need to come up with a better line than that with me." We got hysterical. Was it that funny? Probably not. But we thought so, and laughed, and that's what was important.

BATHROOM HUMOR

We expect to hear toilet jokes from kids and adolescents. Nevertheless, don't be surprised when you hear such humor from a cancer patient; nothing is *verboten*. Cancer patients are totally honest with each other, often more honest than they are with those closest to them. Diarrhea, vomiting, constipation, and urine, (including its color and frequency) may all become topics of discussion. Be prepared, therefore, to hear some vivid intestinal tales. The indignities of treatment are openly discussed. Patients talk to each other and, at times, laugh with each other about the most intimate issues. Dr. Richard Wyatt, a psychiatrist and three-time cancer patient, gave his friend, Jim, some very specific and personal suggestions when Jim was diagnosed with cancer. He recommended that Jim subscribe to extra movie channels to serve as distractions during treatment, but admitted that loss of libido made porno films a waste for him. Describing the problems of constipation, Wyatt recommended Jim keep a supply of disposable enemas in the house. "Just don't leave them in the living room or where the dog can get at them."

In *Prostate Cancer: A Doctor's Personal Triumph*, Bob Fine speaks of the assault on his "ass" during examinations and tests. We might consider this "assault with an anal weapon." Bob was considering options to deal with the aftereffects of his prostate surgery. One possibility was an implant that would have left his penis semi-erect. His wife laughed at that image. He was embarrassed. Not everyone would agree that this was funny, yet he felt it was humorous enough to include in his book.

This toilet story is both funny and sad. In many households there is the eternal struggle between the guy who leaves the toilet seat up and the woman who asks that he put it down when he's finished. This was true for Craig and Karen L., who recently celebrated their 22nd anniversary in Maui. Craig is in a wheelchair because of the effects of cancer. Karen realized how difficult it was for Craig to use the toilet. He had to lift the seat with his foot, and then had trouble bending over to put it down. Karen decided that part of her anniversary gift to him was that she would leave the seat up for him, so he wouldn't have to endure the pain of bending.

CELEBRITIES

Celebrities get our attention. They have the power to inform, teach, cajole, and serve as examples. Celebrities get cancer just like the rest of us. Those who are open about their condition help to save lives. Betty Ford was one of the first to discuss her cancer.

Gilda Radner was able to retain her sense of humor as she documented her struggles with ovarian cancer. More recently, Joe Torre of the New York Yankees, Rudolph Guiliani, former Mayor of New York, and former Vice-presidential candidate Geraldine Ferraro have been direct about their disease and treatment. Their honesty and openness help to demystify the disease and, therefore reduce its terror.

In April 2004, Don Baylor, bench coach for the New York Mets, drove from California to training camp in Port St. Lucie, Florida. He was late for spring training, but this was an important journey for him. A little over a year before, in a routine physical, Baylor was diagnosed with cancer of the blood plasma cells. He underwent extensive treatment, including a stem cell transplant. Baylor, as a major leaguer, had been hit by more pitches than any other player. Yet, he admitted the diagnosis floored him. During treatment, his wife was his mainstay, but he also reached out to Mel Stottlemyre, the pitching coach for the Yankees, who has this same rare cancer. Even major leaguers don't have to go it alone.

Babe Didrikson Zaharias is a major leaguer in the best sense of the word. Considered by many to be the most amazing female athlete ever, the "Babe," in the 1932 Los Angeles Olympics, earned two gold medals in the 80-meter hurdles and the javelin. She also won a silver in the high jump. As a pro golfer, she competed with men in the Los Angeles Open. Dave Anderson, writing recently in *The New York Times*, wrote of her greatest battle against colon cancer. Fifteen months after colostomy surgery, she won her third Women's Open. Her words, if spoken today would resonate as powerfully as those spoken by any of today's athlete cancer survivors—for example, Paul Azinger, Mario Lemieux, and Lance Armstrong. She said, "I want to dedicate at least part of the rest of my life to the job of leading people out of the dark ignorance of cancer. But in the name of Heaven and your own most precious possession, your life, never hesitate about the inconvenience or even the cost of a regular physical checkup. Today, if possible. Tomorrow is too late."

Ruth Handler is known for having created the Barbie doll. Less well known is the fact that she had breast cancer. In the 1970s, there were few prosthetic options for women. After her mastectomy, Handler went to a department store to get fitted. She was disappointed not only in the product but in the way the staff treated her. Frustrated, she founded her own company, Nearly Me. Elaine Woo, in *The Los Angeles Times*, writes that Handler wanted to make an artificial breast real enough so that, as Handler said, "a woman could wear a regular brassiere, stick her chest out and be proud." She did, and then her assistants went to department stores to train sales staffs. Betty Ford was one of her customers. When the actions of others failed, Handler took control and made life more bearable for many breast cancer survivors.

Those celebrities who can make us laugh about cancer deserve special mention. In 1986, Steve Allen was diagnosed with colon cancer. He considered his condition critical, "critical of nurses, critical of doctors, critical of the food, critical of the prices." Richard Crenna, the actor, noticed his voice getting huskier and huskier. Tests revealed a malignant lump behind his laryngeal nerve. Crenna spoke of the importance of a good attitude. His mantra, "This morning I got up on the right side of the grass." Former presidential adviser, Hamilton Jordan, survived three cancers. He writes of his experiences in *No Such Thing As a Bad Day*. He once casually mentioned to a friend that green tea was supposed to help cancer patients. His friend sent 60 pounds of it. Green tea, anyone?

Molly Ivins, the syndicated columnist from Texas, generally uses her caustic humor to write about politics. When she was diagnosed with inflammatory breast cancer, her humor was equally sharp. She calls breast cancer a "no fun" situation. "First they mutilate you; then they poison you; then they burn you. I have been on blind dates better than that."

Erma Bombeck wrote about how kids cope with cancer in *I Want to Grow Hair. I Want to Grow Up, I Want to Go to Boise.* They know how to laugh at their situation. The teenagers had a contest to see who could wait the longest before throwing up after chemo. She tells of a three-year old cancer patient whose hair was starting to grow back. The child looked at her father's balding head and said, "Daddy . . . is your hair coming or going?"

A celebrity doesn't have to have cancer to make a contribution. Rosie O'Donnell and Dr. Deborah Axelrod wrote *Bosom Buddies*, about breast cancer. Dr. Axelrod gives the medical information and O'Donnell uses humor to reinforce the content.

One of her contributions includes this verse,

> *You may think that you're sitting pretty*
> *But here is the real nitty-gritty*
> *You're in for a whammo*
> *If you don't go mammo*
> *Take care of your left and right titty.*

YOUR HUMOR CONNECTION

If you have a long history of friendship, if you're a close family member, if you've worked together for years, and if you are used to talking about sex, marriage, children's problems, basic life issues, then you'll probably have no problem in establishing a climate that will encourage laughter.

Siblings have special relationships. Margie W. had cancer. Her identical twin went with her to the oncologist, who suggested the possibility of a bone marrow transplant. Margie's sister asked the doctor what she had to do to prepare for the procedure. Listening carefully, she looked at her sister and said, "I will give you my bone marrow, a kidney or a piece of my lung or liver, but if you break a fingernail, you're on your own."

Close friends and family can say what casual acquaintances cannot. One woman had a skin cancer, and required extensive facial surgery that included the removal of a large portion of her nose. While she was waiting for plastic surgery and reconstruction, a close friend sent her Groucho glasses and a fake nose. Another woman had a rare cancer of a sweat gland, which presented as a tumor on her lip. Her dear friend said, "Guess this is a message about not sweating the small stuff. Do you think you will learn that lesson from all this?"

Although laughter cannot cure cancer, it certainly can give it a symbolic whack. Chemotherapy does not kill laughter cells; surgery does not cut away one's sense of humor; radiation does not burn away funny memories. Cancer doesn't even improve a patient's ability to tell jokes or make puns. If the patient told bad jokes before chemotherapy, he won't tell better ones after.

Sometimes the humor comes at the strangest times, long after treatment ends. I have a friend who recently made a charitable contribution in my name. When I received the customary letter from the charity, it said, "In memory of Rosanne Kalick." I was shocked for a moment, and then I started laughing. I called my friend and asked her if she knew something I didn't. Sally took the error a lot more seriously than I did. A letter of apology from the charity was quick in coming.

Not too long ago, I went out for dinner with a couple I know well, but not that well. At some point during the meal, Susie started talking about the fact that she had gained weight, and her "boobs" were drooping. For a nanosecond I felt uncomfortable. I no longer have "boobs" to fall. Susie looked at me, realizing her possible faux pas. We both started laughing, she, because she realized I was laughing with her, and I, because I realized she was having this dinner conversation with me as though I had breasts. That's what was great; she had forgotten my surgery. It wasn't that she was insensitive, just that she was thinking of me as whole. When I realized that—and it took only that fraction of a second—everything was fine. Can you always predict when you've crossed the line? I can't say. Try to remember the essence of the person you care about, not what his or her cancer is.

Laughter is a drug of choice. It is free; there is no co-pay. There are no night trips to the drug store. There are no negative side effects. Laughter eases pain. Its supply is unlimited. Laughter is a positive addiction. The dosage, however, must be determined by the patient, not by you. It is the one drug that should be shared once the patient lets the laughter genie out of the bottle. Then, keep laughing.

9

PUZZLE PIECES

What we say may work at one moment and fail the next. What we do one morning may be inappropriate the next evening.

There are puzzle experts, those who can do the Sunday *New York Times* crossword in ink in less than an hour. Others can look at a jigsaw puzzle with hundreds of pieces, and immediately start joining the pieces. For most of us, however, a puzzle takes time, concentration, trial, and error. One of my retirement goals was to learn to complete the Sunday *New York Times* crossword puzzle. I have succeeded on numerous occasions, but never have I done it at one sitting, never in ink, and certainly never without frustration. There are times when I have set the puzzle aside for a few hours, sometimes for a day. Surprise—something then appears that I hadn't noticed before. Leaving the challenge helps me to meet the challenge.

Rabbi Lawrence Kushner in his book, *Honey from the Rock,* uses the image of a jigsaw puzzle as a metaphor for life's relationships and connections. He writes:

> Each lifetime is the pieces of a jigsaw puzzle.
> For some there are more pieces.
> For others the puzzle is more difficult to assemble.
>
> Some seem to be born with a nearly completed puzzle.
> And so it goes.
> Souls going this way and that
> Trying to assemble the myriad parts.
>
> But know this. No one has within themselves
> All the pieces to their puzzle

Like before the days when they used to seal
jigsaw puzzles in cellophane. Insuring that
All the pieces were there.

Everyone carries with them at least one and probably
Many pieces to someone else's puzzle.
Sometimes they know it.
Sometimes they don't.

And when you present your piece
Which is worthless to you,
To another, whether you know it or not,
Whether they know it or not,
You are a messenger from the Most High.

Someone who has cancer is like a puzzle. What words will be fitting to use and when? What behavior is unsuitable? When should we consciously try to interact; when should we back away?

With cancer, certain areas are more puzzling than others, areas for which there are no definitive answers, yet areas to which we must pay attention. If we know some of the complexities, it will become easier to solve.

The worst thing we can do is to run from the puzzle challenge. Diane Cole, writing in *Intouch* magazine, tells of an 80-year old woman who tells her psychologist she wants a divorce. When the therapist asks why, the woman responds that she's been diagnosed with cancer and her husband isn't doing anything to help her. "He doesn't offer to drive me to chemotherapy, to cook dinner, doesn't offer anything. He leaves me alone." The husband later confessed that since he did not know what to do, he left her alone. That's a retreat. I'd like to think the problem could be easily solved by a little communication, but if communication was poor before the diagnosis, it will be a challenge now. Fortunately, since the wife was seeing a therapist, it was a golden opportunity for the therapist to instruct them in communication techniques.

Following are some of the myriad more difficult issues that challenge us. Confront them boldly and fearlessly.

HAIR

Let's assume you see a man who looks as though he's wearing a hairpiece. You are not going to ask him if he's wearing a toupee. If someone you know is undergoing chemotherapy, there will likely be hair loss, often total hair loss. You know that. It is not surprising, therefore, if your eyes gravitate to the hair. However, before you ask the hair question, wait—the patient may bring up the topic. I often spoke about how I hated my wig, how I wore it only when I went outside, how hot it was in the summer, and so on. If the patient wants to talk about what it feels like to be bald, the topic will come up. I have a friend undergoing treatment who wears a wig. It looked particularly good one day, and I asked if she'd recently had it styled. She told me she had had it cut shorter. I didn't feel uncomfortable telling her how good it looked. I wasn't being intrusive, because she knew I knew.

One day, a neighbor, whose name I didn't know, told me how great my hair looked. She didn't know I was wearing a wig. I was tired and perhaps responded too quickly when I said, "It's not my hair; it's a wig. Chemotherapy." The woman just said, "Oh." My response wasn't a good one, but it was a human one. The next time we met in the elevator, I apologized and we had a nice chat. At least she hadn't said, as one patient's friend did, "Is that your hair or a wig?"

It's not just being bald that's so difficult. It's what hair represents in our society. Think of the advertising about hair and hair products. Does your hair have the right sheen? Is it the right color? Are there split ends? Is your dandruff under control? Beautiful hair represents sexuality, virility, youth (how many of us wear our hair gray?). So the loss of hair, literally and emotionally, carries quite a burden.

Margaret felt devastated when she lost her hair. She always wore a scarf or a wig. She felt her hair loss meant she had lost her identity as a woman. It was a while before she let even her husband see her bald. Friends who said, "But it's only hair," or "It will grow again" made her feel worse. Her husband said, "It must really be awful for you." That worked. Margaret needed acknowledgment of her pain. Acknowledgment means the pain, if not totally understood, is at least accepted. Throughout the cancer experience, you'll not likely go wrong if you acknowledge the patient's pain, whether that pain is physical or emotional.

One little girl took a wonderfully humorous approach when it came to her mother's hair loss. She would peep under her mother's scarf and call her "Auntie Fester," a twist on Charles Adams' Uncle Fester. Barbara Stevens in her book, *Not Just One in Eight*, writes of the child whose mother was losing her hair. The child put a positive spin on things; at least she wouldn't get head lice.

Some patients opt to be bald. One woman, a professional speaker who was diagnosed with advanced breast cancer, refused to wear a wig. She worked as much as possible during the chemotherapy, scheduling presentations between treatments. One client, however, insisted the speaker wear a wig, saying ". . . it would draw too much attention to your illness and make the audience uncomfortable if you didn't." Azrieia Jaffe, the author and columnist who specializes in business issues, related the story. Jaffe's friend turned down the speaking engagement. Is there a right or wrong here? I don't know. In a perfect world, it shouldn't make a difference whether the speaker is bald or not. A male who is bald wouldn't have to cancel an appearance. (How ironic the word *appearance* is in this context.) Why should a woman have to cancel one? On the other hand, if the audience were to focus on her baldness rather than on the message, the speaker might not meet with success.

I have a friend who, for years before I had cancer, always ran her hands through my hair after I had it styled. It never bothered me. However, when Sandra's hair began to grow back after her treatments, she felt like a "circus freak" when acquaintances touched her hair. In one day, she heard people say, "Have you had a perm?" "Are you sure your hair has never been curly before?" "I can't get over how curly your hair is." Remember, the cancer patient is vulnerable. What might be laughed off under normal circumstances can be quite upsetting to someone whose entire life is now in turmoil.

When hair begins to grow back, it is often very soft, like a baby's hair. It may be tempting to reach out and touch it. But touch is personal; it can be offensive. Pregnant women often resent when casual acquaintances run their hands over the big belly, and pregnancy is a joyous condition. Cancer patients, too, are often sensitive about intrusion into their personal space.

Mary M. believes we should not joke about hair loss. Her only exceptions are if you also lost your hair, or if you're a very close friend who's joking, and Mary admits that even then the friend might still cause offense. Her sister-in-law sent her a baseball cap. It had medium-length gray hair attached on the sides and bottom. The front of the cap said, "After 40, the only thing worse than gray hair is no hair." Mary cried. What might have seemed funny to someone whose hair was thinning naturally was inappropriate for someone who had lost her hair to cancer.

Most people do not see the patient totally bald since so many patients wear wigs, turbans, baseball caps, or scarves to cover their heads. If the patient feels comfortable with you, he or she may go bareheaded. This can be shocking the first time. Be prepared; it will be easier the next time. As difficult as it is for us to see someone we care about bald, how much more difficult it is for a parent to see his child bald. Claire said, "When my son loses his hair, it makes cancer more real to me. When his hair comes back, I 'think' he's more like his old self, and delude myself to his not being sick anymore."

Alexa R., a four-year old, has something to teach us. Her mother told her that at Thanksgiving, her Grandpa would be bald. She wanted to prepare her child for this dramatic change. Alexa's response was, "That's okay, Mommy. Grandpa's still the same on the inside, right?" Out of the mouths of babes.

We know the obvious things we shouldn't do when it comes to hair loss. Still, in our desire to be sensitive, we shouldn't insult the intelligence of the patient. Judy worked throughout her illness. This meant she had to attend numerous meetings. Her hair was growing back and she decided to go to work without her wig. At one meeting, some colleagues told her how great she looked. At another, no one said a word. "It was bizarre," she said. Think of it. One day, you see your colleague with a full head of hair. The next day, she appears with about an inch or so of hair. How can we pretend there was no change? Being sensitive doesn't mean being oblivious.

Susan wears a wig. She was amazed one day when a casual acquaintance said, "Anything growing under there yet?" We can't talk about hair loss the way we talk about someone's lawn. You can say to your neighbor, "Anything growing under there yet?" when you know he's seeded the lawn. We're not talking about grass here.

The hair loss, the energy loss, the weight loss are all real. We need to remember the real person is still there. If we keep that in mind, we'll do just fine. However, being bald is awful. Depending on the number of treatments, a person can be bald for months. Having lost my hair three times, I can say it never got easier. It's a special kind of pain.

Dr. Bernie Siegel can see someone bald from treatment and turn that emotional pain into a positive. He emphasizes the importance of living in the moment. A patient told him that when her hair grew back, she would do everything she had postponed. Siegel said, "Don't wait until your hair grows back. Do it now, because one never knows what the future will bring. Don't postpone living." Delayed living is risky for all of us.

RELIGION

For some, religion is a particularly difficult topic to consider. Where does religion fit in? The answer is not simple. The guideline may be the same as for the topics of marriage, sex, problems about children, questions dealing with work, and so forth. If you had conversations about religion before the diagnosis, it is all right to continue to do so afterward. However, if you are uncertain of the beliefs of the patient, it is best not to raise the issue unless he does, even if you have strong faith and sincerely want to help.

What continues to work for me generally in the etiquette arena is to ask rather than tell. If I'm visiting someone who is ill, I may simply say, "We have a prayer for healing in which we name those who are ill. May I mention your name at our next service?" Usually, the answer is yes. Most of us in treatment want all the help we can get. What we don't want is to be pressured into prayer. For the patient who's depressed, angry, or in pain, your saying God will take care of him is probably not appropriate. If you say the same thing to someone who is devout, it may be a perfect comment. Know the patient. Diane, for example, is a cancer survivor who has strong feelings about God. She says, "If you're going to be mad at someone because you have cancer, be mad at God. He can take it." You may disagree, but this period is not the time for you to get involved in what could become a major theological disagreement, especially since not everyone believes in God.

There are times when some people may experience a sense of a higher power, even when the situation is not a religious one. Years ago, a colleague of mine was dying of cancer. She was on a respirator. A group of us—Catholics, Protestants, Jews—gathered in a small conference room at the hospital. We began to talk about our friend, Carol R. What I remember was the sense of community we had. Carol's husband was a minister, who led us in a prayer at the end of the morning. Was this a religious experience? I can't say. Did it ease our sadness? Yes. Were we glad we gathered together? Definitely. Did it help Carol? We'll never know.

Chris J. has strong religious convictions. "I am a born-again Christian, very rare in the UK, less than two percent of the population." His belief is that heads he wins, tails he wins. If he dies, he expects to go to heaven. If he lives, that's great. No one would try to take his faith away. No one would ask him why, if his prognosis isn't so great, he still had faith. Why, then, should anyone try to convince a cancer patient who is already struggling through a morass of medical and emotional challenges to accept God? Chris believes that "Recovery from cancer is a matter of calling on all your resources, physical, spiritual, mental, relational and medical." No one would disagree. What we must be careful about is imposing our values, especially our religious values, into the situation.

Nance Guilmartin in her book, *Healing Conversations*, tells how her friend prayed not only for Guilmartin, but also for the doctors, the nurses, and yes, even the equipment. Guilmartin's surgery was on Friday the 13th and the doctor admitted he was using the equipment for the first time. A good time for a prayer.

Bonnie couldn't drive because of severe neuropathy, numbness in her foot. For nearly a year, every Tuesday, her friend would drive home from work, pick Bonnie up, and then the two would go to the weekly Unction, the healing service at their church. She helped Bonnie get to the altar to kneel in prayer. She then insisted that Bonnie and her husband join her family for dinner. This is practicing religion in the best sense of the word. Someone knew how important prayer was to Bonnie, and acted to meet that religious need. Acting religiously means more than talking a good religion.

A religious community can be very helpful. Linda C. calls her church community her "prayer warriors." One of those warriors said she couldn't take away Linda's pain, but she did offer to clean her bathrooms. Linda said, "no," but invited her over for coffee. The woman played with Linda's daughter. In addition, she managed to tidy up, so that the house was spotless when she left. Acting religiously means more than lighting candles.

Michelle tells of those who prayed for her, and those who prayed with her. Her husband prayed out loud every day so that she could hear him. "What I found so touching and so healing to my spirit was that they did what they could. No one did everything, but everyone did something." Not a bad guideline for all of us.

On the negative side, Penny objects to the acquaintances who push what she calls the "Come to Jesus Talks." She does not object to those who say that her husband James is in their prayers. She resents those who say that he has to "accept Jesus Christ as his personal savior, else he won't go to Heaven." Penny interprets their pressure to mean they believe James is about to die. "And the more aggressive people are actually pushing him away from faith, which is not their intention." They have received Bibles, religious medals, and faith-based cancer books that focus on self-healing. Being supportive doesn't mean proselytizing.

Patty's story illustrates the quiet power of religion for some people. Her family business is an auto repair shop next door to a Bible translating office. Mitch, a cancer patient, often repaired the cars of the missionaries who worked there. They would come into the shop to check up on him, to bring small gifts, or just to give a hug. They told him he was in their prayers. Patty says, "We felt as though all of them were our partners. They respected our personal lives and would not pry—just accepting what we would tell them. . . . Quiet love and support was what we received from them." The God issue is similar to other issues. You'll sense whether your help in the religious area is needed or wanted.

THE SCARS

For some, scars from cancer surgery are visible. You may see a voice box or evidence of extensive facial or neck surgery. In most cases, however, the results of cancer surgery are not visible. You won't see the artificial bladder or colostomy bag. Mastectomy scars are extensive, as are the scars from lung surgery. If you are married to someone, or you have a close family member who has had extensive surgery, be prepared for the enormous adjustments he or she has to make to physical change. Those adjustments may take time. Be prepared for some to bare more than their souls to you. They may need you to see them scarred so that you can share in this new reality. Brace yourself; it can be unsettling.

Still, when it comes to asking about the scars, there is a delicate balance. You can't be intrusive lest it appear you have only a clinical interest. David F. has prostate cancer. He feels that some people who ask about the type of cancer are really asking where the cancer is. "If I wanted to tell you where they are going to cut or what they are going to cut out, I would tell you. I think after the surgery I will just drop my pants and show them the scar." He's also been asked how his marriage will fare if he can't sustain an erection. His anger is real, and he is entitled to it.

Many mastectomy patients have no hesitation in undressing openly in the locker room. Others will conceal themselves as much as possible. One of my daughters has seen me without breasts; one has not. I didn't walk around naked in front of friends or family before I got cancer; I don't do so now. If the patient wants you to see the "new look," let her do so. She may need to do this for affirmation of self. There are no rules. *First Look* by Amelia Davis is filled with pictures not of individual women, but of their mastectomies. A brief essay written by the woman accompanies each photograph. These are powerful images.

Jeannie Nash was diagnosed with breast cancer when she was 35. In *The Victoria's Secret Catalog Never Stops Coming*, Jeannie tells of her journey. She has extensive body scars from reconstruction. She even has a new belly button because the surgeon used her body fat to form the new breast. Still, she is willing to show anyone her new breast, "because I want them all to know that I'm not the same."

Elaine Ratner in *The Feisty Woman's Breast Cancer Book* tells about her young daughter's reaction to breast cancer. She had seen her mother's black and blue marks from the biopsy and later the scars from the mastectomy. Her daughter prefers to snuggle with her mother on the "softer" side.

Tell children the truth, but don't overload them with unnecessary information. If they want to know more, they'll ask. Pat's granddaughter asked her if her breast would grow back. It's the kind of question a child would think of. Pat answered her honestly, and the little girl accepted the explanation.

My granddaughter, Maddie, was just four when I had my breast surgery. She came to visit a few days after I came home from the hospital. She had always just run into my arms. Jean, her mother, had told her she shouldn't do that when she visited Grandma that day. Maddie ran down the hall, but when she saw me, she stopped, a few inches in front of me, and began to cry. I couldn't lift her up, so I bent down and hugged her. We walked hand in hand to my apartment. I sat on the couch; she snuggled up, and all was right with the world. Never underestimate the ability of children to adapt to a new situation.

Some cancer scars have profound effects. Philip G. had throat cancer and required a total laryngectomy and reconstruction. He can utter only a few sounds. Imagine spending one's life being able to communicate only by written notes or facial expressions with no hope for conversation. Imagine trying to interact with your children under those circumstances. Imagine Philip sitting for hours and hours watching "in silence and solitude" as his son played baseball. Yet, somehow Philip has been able to communicate with his children.

* * *

This is what he wrote on his daughter's first day at college:

LAUGHTER BY THE MUTE
I had to laugh.
Not an outward bar-room guffaw
Not a lurid cackle
Or even a heaving chuckle
But a quiet exhaling of amused air
An enlivened face and brightened eyes
An inner depth of silent mirth
Heard only by the mute.

Philip has some suggestions for us. He stresses the need for our maintaining eye contact. This is particularly critical given his condition. The patient deserves our total attention. Philip urges that we repeat again and again a variation on the question, "May I help you in some way?" The answer will not always be the same. A refusal at one time may mean an acceptance at another. Telling him he was "going to be fine" were the wrong words. That "hurt so deeply because there is no way I am ever 'going to be fine.'"

Many times, cancer strengthens individuals in ways they never anticipated. Natasha is a good example. She is now in her third year of remission from Stage IIIA Hodgkin's Disease. She was 25 at the time of her diagnosis. She had a one-year-old daughter, and "a no good husband." She claims the cancer gave her the courage to divorce and "never look back."

Scars, visible or not, outline our cancer. They do not define who we are. The National Bone Marrow Transplant Link titles its Emmy-award winning video, *The New Normal: Life After Bone Marrow/Stem Cell Transplant.* Many cancer patients need help in redefining what is normal. It's what they *can* do that's important, not what they can no longer do. The "new normal" may differ in many ways from the old normal. Lance Armstrong, the world-famous bicyclist, knows this. Returning to health wasn't easy. "I was physically recovered, but my soul was still healing," he said.

MACHO MAN

A hockey player is hit by an opponent's stick during a game. He goes off the ice, gets stitched up and returns to play the next period. A football player competes even though his arm is in a cast. Trainers routinely tape athletes' knees, ankles, and wrists before a game. Athletes return to the field days after arthroscopic surgery. It's macho to play hurt. Is Macho Man myth or reality? If Macho Man is a reality, are our expectations for men with cancer different from those for women? Is a man expected to "suck it up" and ignore his physical and emotional pain? How should we speak to the man who can't or won't verbalize about his cancer experience? Should we encourage Macho Man to express his feelings? Will Macho Man be considered a wimp if he joins a support group? Do men react differently from women when it comes to cancer?

The recommendation is that we be as responsive and as sensitive as we can at any given moment, because there are no definitive answers. For instance, don't assume a man will be less upset than a woman when it comes to hair loss. Even though Bill B. was partially bald before he started chemo, he didn't welcome comments such as, "Well, you didn't have much hair to begin with." He chose to shave his head, and later did appreciate the colleague who told him how "hot" he looked that way.

John C.'s 19-year old son humorously played into the Macho Man image. When he saw his father's shaved head, he said, "Whoa, Dad, let's go look at motorcycles."

When John S. lost his hair during treatment, he felt annoyed rather than traumatized. His sons each had different reactions to their father's bald head. The older son, who always wore his hair short, shaved his head in support. The son's employer was startled, but approved of it once he heard the reason. John's younger son, a musician, has long hair down his back. He did not shave his head.

A Californian, John didn't feel traumatized about his hair loss. He knew that a shaved head was not an anomaly. Still, he found his baldness uncomfortable. He was either too hot or too cold. He purchased a beret to wear in the house, a watch cap for bed, and a walking hat for protection from the sun. As he said, "If it's gotta be, at least make it STYLISH." Would a Macho Man have shivered rather than give in to a hat? Some might have, just to be macho. We all know guys like that, don't we?

One young man admits he internalized a lot during his cancer treatment. He didn't want to worry his family. Yet, there were times he did break down, saying, "I don't want to die." At one point, late in his treatment, he was so upset he couldn't even watch the IV going in. One nurse, realizing his anxiety, simply covered the IV with a pillow, so he didn't have to see what was going on. Retrospectively, he believes he should have joined a support group. Even though it's been years since the diagnosis, his fear is reactivated whenever he goes for checkups, especially CAT scans. There isn't a day that goes by without his thinking of his experience. In fact, the illness had so profound an effect on how he sees life that he changed careers and is now an oncology nurse.

Only those closest to Mike K., a management consultant, knew he had cancer. For ten years, he did not "let cancer into the house" or into his workplace. Mike admits that concealing his cancer meant that he had no outlet for his own emotions. On balance, he believes his decision was the correct one. By the time his children learned about the cancer, they were young adults. He told them not only about his illness, but also that during those years he ran support groups assisting others as they dealt with their disease.

Was Mike macho in not revealing his cancer? If he is macho, does Paul lack machismo because he "can't function" if his daughter speaks to him about whether or not she will survive Stage IV breast cancer? Father and daughter are extremely close and discuss most important issues together. A high-level executive, Paul makes important decisions every day, and his daughter respects his opinions. Nevertheless, when it comes to his child, Paul cannot deal with the severity of her illness, or the possibility of a bad outcome.

David S. was only 24 when he found out he had Hodgkin's disease. He had his spleen removed, and then six months of chemotherapy followed by four months of radiation. He was living in Maryland at the time. Maryland is hot and muggy during the summer. David commuted to work and treatment driving his small car that had no air-conditioning. His father had a new full-size air-conditioned car. David considers his father the greatest man he knows.

How did this quiet man deal with his son's illness? He was a man who did not verbalize his feelings. His most direct question was, "Do you need anything?" This father acted. He simply traded cars with his son. There was no need for any involved discussion. The father did what he had to do for his son.

Special attention should be accorded to men who exemplified Macho Men in World War II. Most today are in their seventies or eighties; many are at high risk for prostate and other cancers. They, and most of the rest of us, still think they are heroes from a "good" war. They become particularly sensitive and angry because they never thought of themselves as anything but stoic, indefatigable, and intrepid. As one former Air Force pilot told me, "I cannot ever think of myself as diseased." It behooves us all to be wary, therefore, of men who, when questioned, always respond, "I'm fine."

This attitude makes many of them reticent about reporting pain, or admitting the possibility of illness. And many men who are afflicted become impatient and annoyed with the people who are oversolicitous about their condition. There are certainly younger Macho Men, and their self-appraisals are sometimes heightened by the false bravado of the young.

They may very well refer to themselves off-handedly with a bitter but self-deprecating comment, such as "I won't be able to make babies any more"—or "Well, at least my balls won't get in anybody's way now." But woe unto anyone else who dares to make a remark like that within a Macho Man's earshot!

On the flip side is a man like Hannan W., who has an encyclopedic knowledge of many topics, from boxing to golf, from art to antiques. His need to know served him well professionally, as well as when he was diagnosed with prostate cancer at age 70. His urologist called with the results of the latest biopsy. Hannan "punched the air once," said a couple of "damns," and started on his personal medical journey. Hannan did what more men should do. He called a volunteer hotline and then spoke with survivors from across the country. They discussed treatment options, surgery, seed implantation, and radiation. They talked about how age and health factored into the decision-making. As often happens, once Hannan became public about his condition, others came forward and talked to him about their experiences. His recommendation: we need to be open to all the help and information that is available. Does his approach make him any less macho?

My sense is that male patients, like female patients, will most likely react as individuals, not as types. However, *macho* is a word that may not apply to all men. A football lineman who gets cancer will be just as vulnerable to the physical and emotional aspects of the disease as the rest of us. When it comes to cancer, we cannot think in terms of stereotypes.

THE STRANGER

What should you do if a total stranger begins talking to you about his or her cancer? This happened to Lucy. She was on a cruise, waiting for her husband to join her for lunch. She placed her tray on a table, next to an older woman who was evidently having lunch by herself. After a quick mutual nod, the woman edged closer to Lucy and said, in a confidential tone, "I have cancer." It was a completely startling and unexpected revelation to Lucy, especially since it happened in the midst of what we consider festive vacation surroundings. Lucy reported that she reacted on a purely visceral, instinctive level. She blurted out, "Oh, I'm so sorry! How are you feeling now?" The woman nodded tentatively. To avoid the awkward silence, Lucy surged forth with a barrage of questions. "Are you being treated?" "Where do you go for treatment?" "Who is your doctor?" What became evident was that this woman needed to talk to someone— anyone—willing to engage in conversation about her cancer. The two strangers talked fifteen minutes more. Lucy could tell that the woman felt measurably better for having been permitted to vent her fears, even if it had to be with a perfect stranger.

This type of experience doesn't happen often, but it can. You may be sitting next to someone on an airplane who wants to talk. Most of us pay attention for a few moments and then turn to our book, or our pillow. You may be having your hair cut, and someone strikes up a conversation. You may be waiting for your car's oil to be changed, and someone turns to you. Under ordinary circumstances, we want to get on our way; we do not want to hear about someone we are likely never to see again. However, if a stranger raises the cancer specter, stop, wait, and listen. The woman on the cruise was clearly feeling stressed. Perhaps she had no one to talk to at that time. Perhaps she was at a crossroads in terms of treatment. Whatever the cause, she turned to a stranger and the stranger responded. Should this happen to you, listening may be the most appropriate response after you say something as simple as Lucy's inquiries. Probably, Lucy asked too many questions initially. In that instance, however, asking questions enabled the individual to open up. Once the conversation starts, I wouldn't offer medical advice. Should the stranger become too needy or intrusive, then you may have to retreat. More likely, the individual simply needs a few moments to open up his heart. Consider the experience a gift rather than an obligation. Your presence may really be needed. In this case, it was one woman reaching out to another. Would a man have done the same thing? I'm not sure, but I wonder if a man might feel more comfortable turning to a stranger rather than to a member of his own family. Whatever the reason, if a stranger makes a leap of faith and turns to you, give that person what's needed.

THE TELEPHONE

When I was a young child, we lived in an apartment house that had a dumbwaiter. A dumbwaiter is like a hand-operated elevator. We would put our bags of garbage on it. Ropes moved the dumbwaiter up and down. My best friend lived in the apartment above, and I pulled on the rope to get his attention. He'd put his head out the dumbwaiter opening and we would talk; it was our telephone.

How times have changed. Today, the telephone can be a lifesaver or the bane of our existence. It can be both, often simultaneously, for the cancer patient. Is it all right for you to call? How frequently should you call? When should you call? What should you say? What kinds of questions should you ask? Does it make a difference whether the patient is young or old?

Use your common sense when it comes to speaking to the patient on the telephone. Don't call too early in the morning, or too late at night. I wouldn't call before 10 a.m. or after 9 p.m. If the patient indicates he feels more alert in the morning, that will be your cue. If she says, "I'm a night person; you can call up until midnight," you have your parameter. Generally, keep the conversation short, unless the patient indicates that he wants to stay on the line longer. If you expect the conversation to be substantive or personal, don't make the call from your cell phone on the bus or train.

My friend, Ginette, would call often, and usually the conversation would be short and sweet. "It's Ginette. Wanted you to know I'm thinking of you. Good-bye." Of course, there were many times when we had real conversations. She still has the ability to sound as though she's smiling when she calls. That's something we can all try to emulate. If we sound somber, or overly concerned, then that can have an impact on the tenor of the conversation. Clearly, you don't want to sound flighty or disinterested, but you can sound positive. It's similar to the hospital visit. The call should be something you want to do, not something you feel you are required to do. The patient will sense the difference.

As in all matters of cancer etiquette, listen to the patient. If you have a sense she really wants to have a conversation, stay on the line. Do more listening than talking. If he sounds tired or distracted, say, "I'll call back tomorrow," or "When do you want me to call back?" Even asking, "Is this a good time for you?" can be effective. It is the patient's "call" to talk or not. As with face-to-face conversations, don't ask too many questions, and don't ask questions that are too personal. Consider open-ended questions rather then those that require yes or no answers. Instead of "Are you feeling better today?" try, "How well did you sleep last night?" If the patient has been home for a while, you might say, "I'm going to the supermarket. Do you want to give me a list, or do you want me to pick you up, and you can join me?" "It's beautiful outside. Would you prefer a visit, or are you up for a short walk?"

I can't say when a person will want to engage in a long conversation, and how you define long varies. Personally, even now, I prefer short conversations. Others consider 20 minutes a routine call. Common sense works here as well. A young parent who is recuperating and has young children running around might prefer hearing, "I'd like to take the baby out for a walk this afternoon" to a long chat. On the other hand, an older person who doesn't have many friends or family nearby may welcome a lengthy phone visit. It might be his only contact during a long afternoon. Never underestimate the simple value of the sound of a human voice.

Talking to caregivers may require a slightly different approach. An acquaintance shared the story of his good friend who had to move to Arizona for his wife's health. The wife's cancer is now full-blown. Life is difficult for this couple. The friend calls Arizona weekly. His question is, "What do I say after I inquire about the well-being of both of them? I know he's up to his eyeballs with caring for her and he sounds so morose. I just don't know what to say to him!"

How I wish there were easy answers to this problem, one that occurs all too frequently. This particular telephone problem is compounded, because neither one of the friends can just drop in for a short visit; there is the geographic challenge. The telephone link is the bridge. Here are a few suggestions that might work. What did you talk about when you were face-to-face? Imagine you're still sitting and "schmoozing." Keep a "gyp sheet" of topics and bits of information about the old "neighborhood" near the phone.

Topics could include television—the craze in reality shows, the major crisis on *The Sopranos* or *West Wing*, for example. Certainly, world politics will provoke discussion. Where in the world, literally, is there not a crisis? Sports, especially if it's a guy-to-guy conversation, usually works, particularly if the two men support rival teams. I can only imagine a conversation between a Yankee and Boston Red Sox fan. They would not be at a loss for words. For many, Medicare concerns will work. If it's near election time, talk about the candidates. Recommending and then telling a bit about a current book or movie can be good. What are the children and grandchildren up to? That usually can fill a vacuum. What grandparents don't want to talk about their grandkids?

In this case, both men are lawyers, but only one is still working. They can talk to each other about cases that one has on the docket. Work, office gossip, or a challenge from the job can certainly open up conversation. Depending on your relationship, complaining about your family can help both of you. Weather may sound trite, but if one of the speakers is in Arizona, as in this case, and the other in Connecticut in mid-winter, there will be lots to talk about. Don't forget common interests. It could be the frustration of your golf game, the challenge of the computer, your garden pests. Depending on the individual circumstances, you might want to ask about any support group the patient or caregiver is attending. If you've read a provocative article about the patient's cancer, you could summarize it and offer to mail it. Most important, don't hesitate to say something like, "I really want to stay in touch. I know things are tough now, but you can call me anytime, even if it's just to complain." My last suggestion is that you ask questions that start with the classic, "who, what, when, where or why" words—lead-ins that require more than one-word responses.

THE ORPHANS: RARE CANCERS

A friend quietly tells you he is being tested for mesothelioma. Your mother asks if you know anything about chondrosarcoma. You overhear a conversation in which someone says "cancer" and uses the acronym MEN. What does all this mean?

MEN stands for multiple endocrine neoplasia, a syndrome in which tumors in the endocrine system can develop. Chondrosarcoma is a type of bone cancer that attacks cartilage. Mesothelioma is a cancer often found in the lining of the lung. These are all very rare cancers, often called "orphan cancers" because there are so few treatments, and so few drugs developed specifically for that cancer. If someone you know is diagnosed with a rare cancer, he will face additional difficulties that most other cancer patients will not have to face.

For example, only about 2,300 cases of mesothelioma are diagnosed every year in the United States. With rare cancers, patients may have difficulty finding information. The disease may be very difficult to diagnose, which can mean a delay in treatment. Often, there are few doctors who have expertise with the disease. As a result, the patient may have to travel far for treatment. Since there are few patients in the area to speak with, there will likely be no support group available. When it comes to rare cancers, we must be even more careful about asking too many questions, or about making suggestions regarding consultations, or about making comments as to treatments. It will take the patient with an "orphan cancer" a longer time to absorb the reality of the disease. I can identify with how difficult it is to absorb not only the reality of cancer, but also the reality of having a disease whose name I had never heard before.

AFTERMATH

Time has passed. You've stayed connected. You've given support during the chaos of diagnosis. Treatment is over. The person you care about is recovering, has gained back some weight, is more optimistic, and may even have returned to work. There's no more need to worry about the patient. Right? Wrong.

Patients want to assert their medical independence. On the other hand, they still need support and, as during treatment, often are loath to request it. One incident is still vivid to me. After my second transplant, I came home, knowing I didn't have to return to Little Rock for three months. I wanted some new plants—to symbolize life. Still very weak, I drove to the nursery and bought two of the largest plants they had, a cactus and a fern. I also bought a 20-pound bag of soil. I drove back to my apartment, where Rick, the doorman, loaded everything onto a cart. He offered to take the plants into the apartment for me. I blithely said that that wouldn't be necessary. It took me more than a half-hour to move the two plants across the living room floor. I was sweating with the effort, and was weak for some hours afterward. What I did was stupid. Rick would have been glad to help me; it would have taken him only a few minutes. In my desire to return to wellness, I overestimated what I could do.

Keep an eye on the patient even in his life as a survivor, as someone in remission, as someone who has returned to life. There is no perfect term to use. Patients may overestimate or underestimate their capabilities.

Paying attention, however, does not mean interfering with their efforts.

CELEBRATE LIFE

True, the major pressures are over, but even in remission, the cancer cloud remains. The cancer calendar still goes on. Your role is not over. Cancer calendars need to be written in pencil, but they need to be filled with more than medical appointments. Join with your friend, loved one or colleague as he or she celebrates life. Some transplant patients celebrate second birthdays, using the date of their actual transplant. Many remember the date of their last treatment. If you are a close friend, you may want to jot down those dates to remember them. Whenever I speak to patients who have had cancer, I urge them to plan something special once treatment ends.

A month after my mastectomy, I started chemotherapy that lasted for five months. When that treatment ended, I needed to celebrate life once more. I decided to have my apartment painted—to get a literal fresh start. Some survivors burn their wigs. If we can burn a mortgage, why not a wig? A better suggestion would be to donate the wig to the local cancer center for a financially needy patient. How one celebrates is not important. Join in the recognition that healing has occurred.

How about a wedding? The date was set, when David and Heather heard the shocking news that David had Hodgkin's disease. When David's mother heard the news, she wanted him to postpone the wedding. She said he had to concentrate on his treatments. David was disappointed at his mother's reaction. Heather wanted to keep the date. She had "full complete faith" that he was going to be all right. During the months of treatment, she dragged him to look at flowers, to do what he didn't think he was capable of doing. At times, he wanted to "crawl up and die," but she wouldn't let him.

One can understand the mother's concern and her feeling that the focus had to be on treatment and recovery. One can equally understand the couple's insistence that they get on with their lives, and plan for the future. It's the yin and yang again. Both were right. It's now been more than seven years. Heather and David are married; David's cancer is in remission. They celebrate two anniversaries, one marking the end of treatment, one the date of their marriage.

Only a few will celebrate with a wedding. For the rest of us, the celebration can be a shopping spree, a vacation, a party, retirement, or simply a return to work. Survival needs to be honored.

THE CALENDAR TURNS

The survivor's cancer calendar highlights are often checkup dates. Near the time for the mammography, the PSA test, the CAT scans, or blood work, patient anxiety is likely to increase. Try to be aware of those tests, those dates. The patient may or may not want you to accompany him to these tests. I prefer to go alone. The waiting for results is less traumatic than waiting for the original diagnosis was, but this is still a difficult period. Good results will be another cause for celebration. Setbacks mean the "wagons" will have to circle again. If you're a close friend, you can jot down the dates of the tests on your calendar. This will prepare you for the peaks and valleys of survivorship as they occur.

The cancer calendar is not a perpetual calendar. Patients—permanent émigrés, we hope, from the cancer world—have learned how transitory life can be. That doesn't mean goals still can't be set and met. Our version of long term, however, may differ from yours. If life is a video, some of us might need to fast forward a bit to get to the good parts. Instead of celebrating the 50th anniversary with a big bang, do it for the 40th.

Perhaps patients need to plan more for the short than the long term. My scheduling a trip out of the country in six months is a good goal. My thinking of surviving until my grandchildren's graduations is more of a stretch, but still not unreasonable. You've participated in the pain of the diagnosis and treatment; now it's time to reap the harvest.

Caring responses are meaningful a week after diagnosis, a month after treatment starts, and even when treatment ends. Continuity counts. I used the marathon image to keep me going through lengthy treatment. A friend loaned me a poster of the New York City Marathon, which I kept in my bedroom. Every morning and every evening I saw the runners; I had to keep going as well. Just a poster? Not really.

THE NEW SURVIVORS

Years ago, people would have scoffed at the idea of a National Cancer Survivors Day. There wasn't much talk about survival then. A positive cancer outcome was an oxymoron. Today, however, more and more of us live with, rather than die from cancer. Today, there are now nearly 10 million cancer survivors in the United States, and nearly two-thirds of people with cancer live more than five years after their diagnosis. Does cancer etiquette apply to cancer survivors? Yes.

Some define a survivor as anyone who has been diagnosed with cancer. Others say they are survivors once they complete treatment. Still others wait until they have gone five years post-diagnosis before they use the term to describe themselves. There are those who reject the word entirely. Gina Kolata, writing in *The New York Times*, talks about Dr. Fitzhugh Mullan, himself a cancer patient, who wrote an essay in The *New England Journal of Medicine* nearly 20 years ago, in which he said, "Survival, in fact, begins at the point of diagnosis because that is the time when cancer patients are forced to confront their own mortality." Ellen Stovall, current president and chief executive of the National Coalition for Cancer Survivorship, disagrees. She calls *survivor* an "incendiary" word.

I can understand why there is disagreement over the use of the word. Even though I'm in a good remission from multiple myeloma, specialists still consider my disease incurable. Should I say, "I have myeloma," or should I say, "I had myeloma"? Do I say, "I have breast cancer" or "I had breast cancer"?

Here's where the etiquette comes in. The patient, I think, has the right to say whatever is medically realistic. If the patient is five or more years post-treatment and wants to say he is cured, who are we to contradict him? If another patient says she is living with cancer, rather than she has cancer, isn't that just as reasonable a statement? If a patient simply wants to get on with life and has no use for the term at all, that, too, is all right. Let each patient choose his own definition. The etiquette is to follow the lead of the patient. If he is comfortable with the term survivor, don't argue about it.

The Lance Armstrong Foundation, recognizing the complexity of the issues relating to those who are living long term, is planning to deal with health strategies for cancer survivors. Among the long-term issues survivors face are problems of fertility, sexual dysfunction, stress, and, of course, the constant: the possibility of a recurrence. Other issues of importance are the impact of cancer on an individual's career, or the realization that should a change in employment become necessary, the former patient may be denied health insurance. Relationships can change. Doug Ulman, a survivor of bone cancer and melanoma who is the director of the Lance Armstrong Foundation, stresses the importance of these survivorship issues, saying, "Equal attention has not been paid to quality of life issues that can be significant." On a more personal note, Ulman said, "But what I realized is that there was very little support out there for people who were really thinking longer term about their lives. Not, Will I live or die? But, How well will I live?" In response to these trends, a new magazine, *Heal*, will soon go into publication, and is expected to reach 100,000 readers.

Years ago, in recognition of the reality of survivorship, Richard and Annette Bloch founded the National Cancer Survivors Day Foundation. The Foundation is committed to cancer survivorship issues. The Day is traditionally celebrated throughout the United States, in Canada, and in other countries on the first Sunday in June; 2005 marks the 18th year of this celebration of life. The Day honors not only survivors, but also their health care providers, families, and friends.

When we honor our survivors, we must continue to bear in mind what Gina Kolata said, "But these cancer survivors do have one thing in common. The prospect of death is no longer a cerebral awareness but is an unavoidable part of daily life."

10

Thinking of the cancer, the treatment, the recovery, the checkups, and the prognosis takes up a good deal of space in the patient's life. You can be of enormous help if you find ways to remind the patient that although he has cancer, he is not his cancer. He can still define his life; the cancer should not define him. Here is something you can do with the patient, when the opportunity arises. Have the patient write down what he's accomplished since the diagnosis, what's happened in his new normal life. If she's still in treatment, or if she's still recovering from surgery, it may simply be a walk around the block. It may be that he returns to work, if only part time. It may be that his taste buds are returning, or that a catheter has been removed. Keep and expand the list of these incremental improvements as time goes on. Since I was first diagnosed in 1993, I've traveled to Israel, Morocco, Poland, Mexico, and Italy. I've been blessed with five grandchildren. My third trip to Israel occurred after my transplants. I did the difficult climb up Masada in the pre-dawn hours. It symbolized my new normal.

Although I can no longer jog, I still walk three miles several times a week. I'm still a mother, a grandmother, a friend, someone who loves the movies, fishing, eating ice cream (the light kind), the theatre, music, and other activities. The list goes on. This is part of creating the new normal. It is possible to create new dreams. Thinking of the patient's future, rather than of her diagnosis/treatment/recovery recent past can be useful for everyone.

Patients heal. By focusing on the future, we are less likely to think of the patient as victim. I worry about those who can't even partially lift the cancer veil. Wouldn't it be sadly ironic if the treatment kills the cancer cells, but the patient permits the cancer to take over his soul, so that all he does is study and think about cancer? When does knowledge bring power, and when does it cut one off from the ability to live life? Therein lies the challenge.

Perhaps you remember Harold Russell. He was the disabled World War II veteran who won an Academy Award as supporting actor for his role in *The Best Years of Our Lives*. Russell had lost both hands in the war. He used steel hooks as replacements. Russell died recently, but his words of support for veterans can serve as reminders for all in the cancer story. He said, "It is not what you have lost but what you have left that counts." Remind the patient of what he has, not what he has lost—and the importance of what he does with what he has left.

LONELINESS

How can loneliness be a part of the puzzle? Nurses, doctors, family, and friends often surround the patient. But given today's statistics, we need to acknowledge that many people go through the cancer experience alone. They are the divorced, the widowed, the single, those who are not in a relationship when they get the cancer diagnosis.

I have been blessed with wonderful children and a large community of friends and family. I live alone, and because of that, there are times when I think cancer has a greater power than it might have if I had a partner. If fear strikes, I have no one to turn to at that moment. When the dates for my cancer evaluations draw near, there is no one next to me sharing my anxiety. I am a fairly open person, but I still find it difficult to speak of some of my greatest fears. If the cancer recurs, will I die a painful death? If the cancer recurs, will I be so debilitated from treatment that I'll lose my independence? If the cancer recurs, will I have another chance for remission?

These questions are not unique to me. However, for those who can turn to someone in the middle of the night for reassurance, for those who can ask at almost any time for a needed hug, for those who have someone who still says, "I love you, scars and all," the cancer life may be a little easier to bear. We should give some extra TLC—tender loving care—that extra phone call, that extra effort when it comes to those who face cancer alone. There are many out there who go for treatment alone, who have no one with them at the consultation, who may have to struggle to find someone to be there for the surgeon to talk to after the operation. This is another part of cancer reality, another piece of the puzzle.

THE THERMOSTAT

We know that the patient faces huge emotional and physical challenges. If we cannot control our anger, our fear, our angst, we are more likely to say or do the wrong thing. We need to recognize our own emotional thermostat. My daughter, Jean, is honest enough to admit that she was "pissed off a lot" about my cancer, especially the second time around. She wasn't as frightened as the first time, because I had recovered so well from the two transplants, but she was terrified during my breast cancer surgery. Jean said that when I "ditched" the wig, she felt she had her mother back. Her strength was not only in being there for me, but in being honest about her own emotions.

The patient's thermostat will give you some clue as to the progress of his or her recovery. One simple sign may be when she prepares a special meal. It may be when he walks the dog for the first time. Forcing recovery will be counterproductive. No one wants to recover more than the patient. During the recovery period, the patient's fear is likely to fade in and out. Perhaps ten or twenty years from now, I'll think less about my cancers, not yet. You need to remember the ebb and flow of cancer fear.

Be careful about how you express your emotions in front of the patient. Watch the patient's thermostat as well as yours. Expect variations. In *The Human Side of Cancer*, one patient who has recurrent lung cancer says, "One day I go shopping like crazy and buy new clothes and plan a thousand things to do. The next day, panic sets in, and I start cleaning out my closets and giving everything away."

Earlier, I told of the mother who sent a sympathy card to her daughter when she was diagnosed with cancer. Talk about a thermostat out of control! Lillie Shockney, Director of Education and Outreach for the Johns Hopkins Breast Center, updated that story. The mother was recently diagnosed with lung cancer. The daughter asked Shockney for advice. Shockney's response, a wonderful one, was that she could send her mother a sympathy card, or she could provide support. The daughter chose support and became her mother's caregiver. Not surprisingly, the mother apologized to her daughter. At least if we acknowledge the vagaries of the thermostat, we will be less surprised or disappointed when the temperature changes.

SILENCE

Silence can be a negative or a positive. Maggie's son had Hodgkin's lymphoma. Certainly, there are fewer pains greater than having to watch one's child undergo cancer treatment. We must be particularly sensitive in such an instance. Sadly, one of Maggie's friends ignored her during this stressful time of her life. That ended the friendship. This is the negative power of silence.

Silence is more often a positive. Norman Stanton, a minister, believes that silence can be an important "presence." He believes that one reason people stay away is "They can't imagine what they would say that would be appropriate. In fact, what they say is not the issue. It is that they can be with the person. . . . Above all, it is about communicating to the person that they are thought of, valued, wanted, enjoyed, etc." This, we can all do.

Words are not always necessary, but listening is. If we're listening, we're not speaking. If we're listening, we should be listening totally, not necessarily thinking of a response to what we're hearing. This listening/ silence is not the same listening we do at a committee meeting.

Mark exemplifies the power of positive silence. He consistently visited Carrie in the hospital, usually in the evening. When he was there, Carrie's parents could go out for a cup of coffee or dinner. She says, "Mostly he would just sit there and 'be' in the room. His presence was more important than his words. What made his presence even more of a gift was that Mark is "needle/blood/hospital/phobic." She contrasts his presence with two other friends who came every day, but their major activity was fighting with each other. There's being there, and there's being there.

In the movie, *Amadeus*, the king said that Mozart's music had too many notes. Sometimes we have too many words. Don't worry too much about your words. Your presence is what really counts. If words need to be spoken, you and the patient will find them. I don't know whether the need for constant speech is peculiar to our culture or not, but we seem to be uncomfortable with silence. Silence is not always a vacuum that has to be filled. In cancer time, silence may provide a quiet zone, a place where, for a few moments at least, cancer cannot enter. What better affirmation can there be than for two people to be together and know that nothing has to be said? Even if you're just sitting together watching an old movie, you're still bonding.

US

Imagine yourself trading places with the patient. What would you want people to say or do for you? We need to step back at times and look at ourselves. Are our emotions interfering with our relationship? Which fears are stopping us from doing our best? What memories are clouding our judgment? Knowing our own frailties can prevent us from speaking or acting inappropriately. Acknowledging our anger at the situation can be helpful. Howard is suffering badly. His friend, Lori says, "Right now I'm mad . . . mad that they can't figure out how to fix this. Mad that this sweet, kind, brave man has to go through this. Just MAD." She admits she's also sad and scared.

I don't think we speak enough about our reactions as friends, family, and colleagues. We need to have a venue where we can share our emotions. I doubt a support group would turn anyone away, but support groups tend to focus on the patient and on the immediate family. Should we speak to the patient about how *we're* feeling? Should colleagues or friends speak among themselves? Should we do both? Can there be a support group for those indirectly affected by cancer? I have no answers, but the first step is to raise the issue.

There are times I would have welcomed hearing my friends and family speak to me about how they felt about my situation. Words can signal that you care. If you speak, then the patient will also have a chance to say how angry, sad, and frightened *he* is. Knowing how much or how little to say is difficult. Still, if we admit our feelings, we can understand them better.

If we don't admit our emotions, they may haunt us in the future. Tom's brother was a young man when he died. Tom had young children. His life was a busy one. He spent time with his brother, but years later, Tom still felt guilty, thinking he hadn't been with his brother enough at the end. Others have told me that they feel guilty because they did not attend their friend's funeral, or because they didn't invest enough in the friendship during the critical cancer period, or they didn't visit enough. Perhaps it's human nature to look back with regrets. I think, though, that the more we do, the more we admit our love, the more we are present, the more open we are, the fewer regrets we'll have later on.

There's no question that you want to do something, anything to make things better. I know that when I want to do something for someone, it's also related to my own feeling of helplessness for this person I care about. If possible, this is something you and the patient may want to speak about.

As a patient, I hated to ask for any kind of help. I accepted it only when I absolutely had to. I am learning only now that if I permit my friends to help me, I'm helping them as well.

Attitude can hurt. Kim's five-year old daughter has cancer. Another mother said she wanted to get a gift for the child. Kim indicated that her daughter had plenty of toys and didn't need any more. The mother admitted that she *really* wanted to do this for her own daughter, to teach her daughter to be kind. Kim's internal response was, "Grrrrrr . . . don't let us get in the way of your philanthropy." Was Kim overreacting? Perhaps, perhaps not. Kim may have resented the fact that her daughter was being made an object lesson. The other mother was manipulating the situation to satisfy her own needs. This incident illustrates how sensitive even the caregiver is when it involves the needs of the patient.

In October, Jane B. told a friend of her cancer diagnosis. The two lost touch for several months. Some time after Christmas, Jane's friend wrote to her, "I cannot possibly believe you have anything like cancer . . . so my advice to you is to get your act together, lose some weight, have your hair restyled and go and have a good time in a warm climate." Unbelievable! Why would anyone say she has cancer if she doesn't? What prompted this person to make such a statement? What was her emotional baggage? Jane suggested that this woman was so afraid of cancer, she literally tuned out the message. Pointers on cancer etiquette will probably not help someone like that.

Shirley T. speaks of the givers and the takers. The takers stay too long, ask thoughtless questions, say the wrong thing. She was brought to tears when someone asked her, "What does it feel like to lose your hair?" If she wanted to talk about what it felt like, she would have raised the issue. I wouldn't blame Shirley for saying, "What do you *think* it feels like?" On another occasion, this same thoughtless person remarked that Shirley looked good, except for her skin. "I can tell the chemo has ravaged your skin." If we would stop to think about trading places, we may wisely change our selection of words.

THE LITTLE C'S

Instead of focusing on "The Big C," try focusing on "little C's." These are connection, community, compassion, and commitment. If we think of the power of the "little C's," "The Big C" may have less power over us. As a connecting link, you can encourage the patient to think of life after recovery. What does he want to give back to those who have supported him during his cancer experience? Dick, a cancer survivor, taught me about the "little C's." He told me of his volunteer work on a hotline. I called The Bloch Cancer Hot Line in Kansas City, founded by Richard and Annette Bloch, and signed on as a volunteer.

When a newly diagnosed patient calls the hotline, he or she is paired up with someone of the same sex, close to the same age, who has a similar cancer. The volunteer does not give medical advice, but clearly represents someone who has been down a similar path. The "newbie" can speak openly and get some of his questions answered. Richard Bloch was one of the founders of H & R Block. Years ago, he was diagnosed with terminal lung cancer. He beat the odds and survived many years following his treatment. He and his wife felt that by creating this helpline, he could help others facing cancer. I also volunteer for a hotline for the International Myeloma Foundation, and the NBMTLink (the National Bone Marrow Transplant Link). These organizations supply e-mail addresses as well as phone numbers to people who need to learn about their disease. Thus, the "little C's" provide power to the patient.

NOTHING BUT THE TRUTH

When is the truth not the truth? If the truth is too painful, should it be withheld? If you tell most of the truth but not all, are you lying? Cancer truth brings pain. For example, "You'll need surgery." "I can't guarantee you won't be impotent." "You'll need a permanent colostomy." Physicians must tell patients the truth about their condition. The issues are how much truth needs to be told at any given time, and how to tell it.

I've always been honest with my children. They read every word of the protocol for the two stem cell transplants I received. Telling the truth is part of our relationship. When it came to the breast cancer, I told them most of the truth, but not all of it. That was a mistake.

The additional mammographies I took indicated cancer in both breasts. Biopsies confirmed the diagnosis. At the time, both daughters were pregnant. I told them I was having a biopsy, not that I was having two biopsies. There was still a chance that one breast might be free of cancer. My thinking was that they should not have to worry about two mastectomies. If a second mastectomy turned out to be unnecessary, I would have given them needless anxiety. As it turned out, I did need the double mastectomy. Jean went into labor the day I got the biopsy results. I had to tell her soon after she gave birth. I would have waited, but her first question to me was about the biopsies. To this day, I wonder if I did the right thing by clouding the truth in the first place.

Generally, I think it's best to tell the whole truth as soon as possible. It will prevent getting lost in half-truths down the road. It will provide the basis for decision-making. It can set the climate for open discussion.

We may question how doctors tell the truth, but they are honest, and they represent the medical interests of the patient. Richard Bloch's wife, Annette, asked the doctor to step outside Richard's room so she could speak with him. The doctor strode back into Bloch's room with Annette and scolded her in front of Richard. "He told her never to ask him a question about me except in front of my face. There could be no secrets from a cancer patient if there was any hope that the patient could get well."

Think of the implication of that statement. As a cancer patient, I know I have one of nature's worst diseases. As a cancer patient, I am afraid that the disease will metastasize. I worry that any fever, an inability to urinate, the most minor rash can indicate a serious problem. If I think others have more information than I, my cancer fantasies will grow. If I know the truth, I can deal with it. What is hidden can only frighten me more. Here the cancer patient is like a child who is frightened during the night. We need someone to turn on the lights. The cancer monster will not disappear, but at least we can see and face it.

In some cases, however, the patient may say, "I don't want to know the details. Just tell me what I have to do." That perspective too must be respected. If the patient wants his closest relative to be the cancer buffer, so be it. In *The First Look*, Amelia Davis tells of how Maxine's doctor informed her husband that the breast cancer would probably spread to his wife's lungs. Her husband didn't tell Maxine for 33 years. Was he wrong? We can't make that judgment. Generally though, we should give the patient as much information as she or he can absorb. Those who don't want to know at one time may want to at a later date.

Truth also affects communication between the patient and his friends and family. You want me to be upbeat. The patient who seems like a good fighter gets praise. Being negative is tolerated, but not for long. You'll let me cry, but how often and for how long? I wonder whether, if we allowed more leeway in speaking the truth of the emotional side of cancer, the power of cancer would lessen. Will I still be loved even when I cry? Will I be abandoned if I show my anger at getting a second cancer? Will you still visit if I don't laugh? If I break down, will you see me as permanently broken? The etiquette is in accepting the reality both of the disease and of the person's reaction to the disease. Understanding the emotional power of cancer may promote healing, because it means you accept the patient, warts and all.

THE ROAD TAKEN

Most of us rubberneck at the sight of an accident. If it's a serious enough crash, we may gasp, or at the very least drive carefully for a while. How many miles does it take before the accident image fades, and our foot goes down a bit heavier on the gas pedal? Within a short time we're focusing on the road ahead, not on what we've seen on the road behind.

Cancer takes us on a different road. The cancer survivor, if he doesn't change direction totally, at least now checks the map more carefully. Often he does change the route. This reevaluation may prove helpful to all of us. Do we need to celebrate life more? Are we running to too many activities? Where are our life connections weakest, strongest?

You can run, but you can't hide. At some point, you'll have to face the fact that you or someone you care about will have cancer. If we care now, if we become sensitive to the needs of others, if we monitor our behavior during this trying time, our relationships will strengthen. We will be part of the healing solution.

11

CARING FOR THE CAREGIVER
24/7

The cancer story is primarily the patient's, but a significant part of it involves the primary caregiver. That person may be a spouse, a significant other (remember the grateful praise former Mayor Rudy Giuliani heaped on Judith Nathan when he endured prostate cancer), a relative, or a dear friend. If you're not a caregiver now, chances are you will be someday, or you have been already. John Langone, science writer for *The New York Times*, reports that 25 million Americans are caregivers for those who are seriously ill.

We can only imagine how difficult it must be for the caregiver who has a 24/7 schedule. Responsibilities, usually shared, may now be totally transferred to him or her. Financial pressures intensify when two incomes become one, even if only temporarily. Children still need the care and attention of parents. The caregiver often has to play the role for two. It may even be necessary for him to physically contend with the patient's discomfort from debilitating treatment, and it is usually the caregiver who provides distraction to counter the patient's changing moods.

We need to hear their problems, their anger, their fears, their frustration, their pain. We need to be prepared to act in their interests as well as those of the patient. They, too, need kind words and attention. Their stress and pain, although different from the patient's, are very real, nevertheless. Supplying literal and emotional breaks for the caregiver will be a great act of support. What we don't want to do is to treat the caregiver like a "ghost," which is how one caregiver said she was made to feel. People asked about her husband's health, but ignored her totally. So, lend an ear.

We need to listen to what the caregiver says or doesn't say. One man's wife, with stage IV colon cancer, spent hours working on her insurance problems, and every month there seemed to be more and more such problems. When she had a fall, her husband did not report it to the nurses, but he did continue to complain to the staff about her insurance issues. Staff members felt that his focus on the billing was his way of denying the severity of his wife's illness. If we sense the caregiver is focused too much in one area, we can look more closely into what's going on. If he or she seems particularly upset, we may need to tell his adult children or some other close family member to take note of what's happening. We may have to participate more actively in the situation. Our emotional antennae will prove useful here.

Peg received a phone call from a woman inquiring about her husband's condition. When she started crying about her husband's prognosis, the woman told her she needed a "better attitude." Peg felt that was a cruel response. The woman may have thought she was serving as cheerleader, but she certainly failed to help Peg. Our role with the caregiver cannot be a judgmental one. It is not our call to say, "Oh, you're overreacting," or "Be strong." Our role is to give support in any way we can. Later, this woman sent two get-well cards to Peg's husband. Peg felt slighted because her name wasn't on the envelope as well. This may be a gentle reminder for all of us: if you send a card or note to the patient, think about adding regards or a postscript for the caregiver.

If the patient's illness, unfortunately, is terminal, the agony and the burdens of the caregiver clearly mount. Even during the last months of Mack's life, Ina encouraged him to do as much for himself as possible. When he began to overmedicate himself, Ina had to take responsibility for the scheduling of his medicines. She had to continue to work, but she worried constantly. Would he fail to turn off the burner on the stove? Would the water in the sink run continuously? If he didn't respond to her calls from the office, she hurried home to check on him. This is only a snapshot of what some caregivers face.

Occasionally, the dynamics of friendship can change under the stress of illness. Jo Ann was shocked when her very good friend got mad at her, angry enough to end the friendship, simply because Jo Ann had not called to give her the latest blood test results. Wasn't this friend being overbearing? Yes, but you don't know how you would react to overwhelming concern for a dear friend. We need to focus not on our reactions to the cancer, but on its effects on the people we care about. Jo Ann lost not only a friend but also a potential caregiver.

One caregiver, Danna Syltebo, suggests that people not ask about how she, the caregiver, is doing. "I will tell you how she is doing; she is doing lousy. She is tired, she is overwhelmed, she is sad, she is scared, and she is guilt-ridden for hoping the nightmare will not last forever." She probably won't say that if you see her in the parking lot though. She suggests you say how glad you are to see *her*. And, if that comment were followed by suggesting you grab a cup of coffee together, it would be even better. Little things mean a lot.

At all times, try to honor the patient's and the caregiver's requests. Encourage whimsy. If it's a warm night, and your friend wants to walk in the rain, try to do it. If he gets an urge to go to the shore, find out if the doctor will give an OK, and help the family make the plans. One of the few times I was alone in Little Rock, I decided I needed a movie. It was only a few blocks to the mall; still, it was a great effort. I had to wear a mask because I was neutrapenic. Someone asked me if I had serious allergies and I said, "Yes." I enjoyed the movie and my few hours of the non-cancer life. Whatever the patient can do for himself is beneficial for everyone, including the caregivers.

Marissa A. is a caregiver who suggests that people not "compete with grief." If she says she is tired or worried, it should not be taken as an invitation for others to tell long, convoluted tales of the problems in their lives. What the caregiver needs, she says, is an "open heart"—someone who is able to listen, someone who is welcoming without words.

What we can do is give the caregiver more than an isolated hour or two. We can schedule time, individually or in concert with other family and friends, so that the caregiver can take a deep breath and inhale life for himself. Maybe he needs a round of golf, or a few sets of tennis. Maybe she needs time for a haircut, a massage, a manicure, or even just a hot bubble bath. Wandering through the supermarket for a caregiver, unrushed by the need to get home quickly, can provide welcome relief. Peg uses a wonderful metaphor for this. In an airplane emergency, people are urged to start their own oxygen before attempting to help others. "You can't help anyone if you aren't getting oxygen yourself." Our job is to see that the caregiver's oxygen supply is never threatened. He is the most vital element in the non-medical life of the patient.

When a parent with young children has cancer, a caring community will be critically important. First, however, the parents have to set the parameters. Children should be told only as much as they can process, intellectually and emotionally. Mary has an aggressive form of cancer. Mary and George, her husband, knew they had to deal with the reality that their two children might grow up without a mother. Jack was seven and a half years old and Anne only seven months old when their mother was diagnosed.

Jack, who is very close to his mother, was aware of what was happening. Mary and George chose to tell him that his mother was very ill and would not be able to run, jump, and wrestle with him as she had done. Now, Jack focuses on his mother's good days. Using his imagination, Jack has created a world and mythology of the Cancer King. He draws comics to illustrate this world. Anne knows her mother goes to the doctor frequently, and that her mother cannot pick her up; but she also knows that they can still snuggle together.

Clearly, under these circumstances, one caregiver cannot do everything. Here's where the caring community comes in. George reached out to his family and community. Neighbors and church friends help with the basic tasks of shopping, meal preparation, and babysitting. Carefully selected paid helpers spend a good deal of time with Anne, in particular; she knows she is loved. Prayer groups give religious support. The caregivers take their cue from Mary and George. The children consistently hear words of truth from their parents, and everyone else who is involved in this network. These are supportive groups working in tandem, not "fractionizing," as George put it.

THE COATS

With the 24/7 schedule so many caregivers have, on occasion a misstep can occur. One man described by the patient as "a saintly caregiver" sustained his role for more than 20 years. He was this woman's only life support.

When she had a rare moment of "wellness," Harold liked to take his wife shopping. He knew she enjoyed wandering through the shops looking at clothes.

On one of those outings, Sophie glimpsed a beautiful coat. It was lovely, but costly. Still, she decided to buy it. Her "saintly caregiver" stopped her cold, saying, "You can't buy that. You won't live long enough to get your money's worth out of it." Stung by his words, Sophie said nothing; she quietly hung the coat back on the rack.

For those few seconds, even this most devoted, dedicated caregiver, failed Sophie with his ill-considered remark. He succeeded only in hurting his wife. For years, he has regretted those words. Later, he realized that in that store, at that moment, being practical was very impractical.

When she smiled with joy at the beautiful coat, he should not have brought up the issue of price. He simply should have said, "Go for it." Her joy in owning and wearing the coat, no matter how short the time she had left, would have been well worth the price.

Certainly there will be many occasions when patients and caregivers need to watch their finances. Occasionally, however, it may not "pay" to be sensible. Sophie missed out on the occasions when she could have walked proudly in her coat. The bottom line should have been the value of the coat to the patient, not the cost of the coat. This fiscal decision strained the bond between these two people who cared so much for each other.

My sense is that we should offer as many opportunities as possible for the patient to be spontaneous. Let the patient do the less than traditional— to buy the quirky shirt, go to the doubleheader, splurge on a weekend trip. At the very least, there will be a positive memory at the end of the adventure. At most, the patient will feel rejuvenated, ready to get back into the fight against the cancer. True, dollars can be misspent, but who among us has not done that? Even the caregiver can err. We want to create positive moments, not regrets.

In contrast to the coat that was never purchased is the story of the man who bought a mink coat for his wife, because he knew she had always wanted one. They both knew they wouldn't get their money's worth out of it. She wore it proudly for six months.

ONE CAREGIVER'S STORY

Without question, the caregiver's job is complex on many levels. Through a friend, I learned of an extraordinary, private e-mail journal kept by a husband whose wife needed a mastectomy. In the hope that his journal would provide valuable insights for other caregivers, he has given me permission to quote from his many postings to relatives and friends that covered more than a year.

Ted chose e-mails as the best way to communicate with friends and family about the status of Lois's breast cancer. The first e-mail went to 29 recipients. It gave the date of her surgery, the name of the surgeons, the name and address of the hospital, and the hospital phone number.

The e-mails soon expanded from a simple update on Lois's condition to what was happening in the family, to their reactions to the chaos of cancer, to Ted's concerns about his interactions with his wife. The computer connection created an emotional community center for everyone on the list. Ted knew instinctively to include information about Lois as her own woman, not merely Lois, the cancer patient. For example, he reports that Lois sent flowers to the wives of her surgeons, a "classic" Lois gesture. Her surgery and reconstruction took place on Valentine's Day and would continue through the evening. She knew that at least one of the doctors would not be home to celebrate with his wife. Thanks to Lois, his wife would have flowers.

Within a few weeks, the list grew to more than 50 names. The correspondents learned that Lois's surgery lasted nearly eight hours; that the plastic surgeon didn't finish until 10 p.m., that she didn't leave the recovery room until after midnight. Ted told his list that Lois was already telling him and the nurses what to do and how to do it. He was giving the facts, and the most critical fact was that Lois was still Lois.

Ted well knew the importance of staying connected. He told the group that Lois's sister would be with them for several days and that her "most tenured" friend would be there to give support the following weekend. He knew the value of those on the list. He knew the value of their every kindness, from those who would walk the dog to those who would do the driving. Everyone's goal was to get Lois back "to where she belongs."

Ted, knowing Lois does not easily obey orders, stayed "neutral" on the question of when Lois could see her friends. He wanted to listen to the professionals who suggested she wait, but he was smart enough not to get "in between Lois and her preferences."

It was Ted, Lois, family, and friends. Ted never let the cancer stop their world. He told everyone that their children left a few days after their mother's surgery to go on a 60th anniversary cruise for Ted's parents. Neither Ted nor Lois considered asking the kids to say home. They knew that although cancer snapshots would become a part of the family album, the album needed snapshots of life beyond cancer.

One of Ted's messages read, "Group hug NOW." This occurred when Lois got a clean pathology report. Though the news was great, Lois was feeling lousy. He asked her to smile at the news. She showed him "1.4 seconds of 4.5 teeth." He suggested she try to forget for a few seconds that she was nauseous. "Sure, you're not the one who's nauseous", she responded. Ted continued, "She didn't take any calls, spent only three minutes with her three visitors and her conversation with me was limited to 'don't talk,' 'don't touch me,' and similar affectionate phrases."

Ted often had to restrain himself. He was feeling positive, but he had to be sensitive to Lois, who was having terrible days. Here, Ted's instincts were good. Lois was not able to assimilate information at that time. If Ted had urged her to be more positive then, it might have been too stressful for both of them.

Things did improve. Ted expected Lois to ask about getting back on the tennis court, and to make plans for going out to dinner with friends. However, Lois continued to have pain, nausea, and severe headaches. She developed rashes and adhesions. Ted kept his feelings to himself, not out of a lack of concern, but because he knew she had the right to feel lousy.

Then, Ted told the group to get ready because Lois, with her "killer overhead," would soon be back on the court. Still, Ted could admit his own anxiety even though things were going well. He attributes this anxiety to his "erratic estrogen levels." While the doctors were considering treatment options, Lois and Ted made a gutsy decision. Five weeks after the surgery, they decided to take a previously booked trip to Rome for a long weekend to an academic conference Lois wanted to attend. The doctors gave the medical thumbs-up. The Rome adventure worked. Only a few of the attendees even knew that Lois was recuperating from major surgery.

In one e-mail, Ted informed the group of the treatment options. Three oncologists offered their plans; there were some differences as to what would be the best protocol to follow. Once Lois made her decision, Ted told the group who the oncologist was, the drugs to be used, and the length of the treatment. The group, by popular demand, insisted that Ted continue his e-mails even though Lois's surgery and recuperative period were over. They wanted to stay connected during the chemotherapy as well.

Ted reported that Lois had nausea, fatigue, and anxiety from the treatment. She developed a severe cold that lasted three weeks. She lost some sense of smell and taste. Still, she managed to get to a movie, play a bit of tennis, and socialize with friends. Innocently, Ted mentioned to her that although a temporary loss of one's sense of taste and smell must be annoying, it's not that important in the larger scheme of things. Lois's response: "That's easy for you to say. What the hell do you know? You'll eat anything anyway."

Clearly, Lois knows she can say whatever she wants to Ted. He, however, must be careful of what he says. Even the caregiver—perhaps especially the caregiver—must know when to speak and when to be silent. It's almost as though there's a verbal seesaw, with Lois on one side and Ted on the other. Ted's optimism cannot always balance the physical and emotional burdens Lois is carrying. "She cried herself to sleep last night, telling me how much she hates these infusions, doesn't want to do this next one, etc." Lois says, "I feel lousy all week, and then when I start to feel almost human, I go to the doctor, and they give me this stuff that I know will make me feel lousy all over again. I hate it and I don't want to do it!"

What should the caregiver do when the patient is weak physically and emotionally? Ted's response may work for many. He does not come out with a cliché such as "Buck up." He acknowledges Lois's feelings. He knows not to try to talk her out of what she is feeling. He puts it this way: "Unfortunately, she is correct and I have nothing intelligent to say in response. I just shut up and hope that the morning brings enough renewed resolve to get her through the day. So far, it always has."

Even though Lois is still in treatment, Ted makes plans for them to travel to the wedding of Lois's dear friend. Life transcends chemotherapy— an important lesson for all of us.

Side effects continue. Ted learns what many of us who have had treatment know. "Normal" chemotherapy side effects are difficult. But as Ted writes, "There is no reserve of physical strength to do the daily battles that we usually can handle." In spite of the difficulties, Lois and Ted remain optimistic. "We plan to be much more than survivors; we plan to be thrivers."

At one point, Ted felt particularly optimistic. He thought he knew Lois and her situation quite well. He was wrong. "THE SIN OF PRIDE," he wrote. "Last night she cried herself to sleep, saying that she hates this, she may not go to the doctor today, she might not go to France on Wednesday, etc. I understand NOTHING. Hopefully with the dawning of a new day, she will call up her reserves of emotional strength, as she has been doing, get into NYC, and face the poison one more time. I think that I'll call home now and find out how I am wrong again! Every day is a new adventure. The only thing that is consistent is that I don't know squat!!"

Some of Lois's responses to Ted's encouragement are unprintable. He understands that reality when Lois admits her fears about recurrence, about the long-range effects of the chemo, about the five years of Tamoxifen she must take, about her failing taste buds, and about the myriad other fears a cancer patient has; he knows he should say as few words as possible. Sometimes it is best for the caregiver to listen. Ted accepts that and doesn't try to minimize her concerns. He chooses to focus on how far they have come in seven months.

There is no instant recovery. No one ends treatment and is immediately transformed from a cancer patient to a survivor/thriver. Some make the transition quickly; others need many weeks or months. Ted realizes the path can be circuitous. Knowing his wife's many strengths, he readies for her dynamic return. He compares her to a tornado, "powerful, unpredictable, independent, leaves a mess in its path, but fun to watch." It is probable that this internal energy gave her the power to persevere.

The recovery tornado took Lois and Ted to France. Lois painted. French wine enhanced their "spirits" in more ways than one. Once home, Lois began to play more tennis. She began to cook. In reporting these positive changes, Ted consistently adds his thanks to the e-mail group for their prayers, thoughts, and support.

Ted can serve as one role model for caregivers. We want any caregiver to do as Ted did: he gave us the information we needed, information about Lois, himself, and the family. He comforted us as best he could. At times, he even had to give support to his supporters. At one point, some in the e-mail group thought he was slanting the reports. "Honestly, I have tried to be as 'straight' as possible; no excess drama and no sugar," Ted wrote. Still, the caregiver's primary responsibility is to the patient. It is to Ted's credit that he was sensitive to the needs of friends and family; however, we need to be reminded that we must get our comfort and strength from each other, not from the caregiver. What neither the caregiver nor the patient needs is an additional layer of responsibility, to think cancer is having a negative effect on us. Ted's e-mails teach us that the cancer life and the noncancer life are parallel. We need to accept that parallelism.

One evening, Lois attended an American Cancer Society program for patients, "Look Good . . . Feel Better." She came home wearing a wig. When Ted saw her in the wig for the first time, he wasn't sure how to react. It was a "kick" for him to see her so enthusiastic. But if he was too positive, would Lois think he thought she looked terrible with thinning hair? If he didn't share her joy, momentary as it might be, would he be a "killjoy?" What was the right response? Probably there is no one right response. Ted felt good about his interaction with Lois that evening. Ted's story confirms that even the caregiver will not always know what to say or do. When the caregiver faces such moments and turns to us, our job is to be sensitive, and to offer a receptive ear and heart. At those times, we can serve as sounding boards.

During the cancer year, an unexpected roadblock slowed Lois's progress. She developed two hernias, which may have resulted from the breast reconstruction surgery. The hernia surgery was more complicated than they had anticipated. Ted and Lois had to adjust their timetable. Their new target date for closing the official cancer calendar was Valentine's Day, one year after her breast cancer surgery.

Lois became more emotional as the months went on, possibly as a result of the stresses of the unanticipated surgery, residual effects from the diagnosis, and the side effects of chemotherapy. Like many cancer patients, she wanted to will herself to heal more quickly than her body was able. Like many cancer patients, she was angry, and this made her more volatile with those around her. She turned her anger toward the person closest to her, Ted. During this time, it was important that Lois schedule regular activities such as tennis practice to give her a raison d'être for getting out of bed in the morning. It was then that Lois began seeing a psychiatrist.

It is not unusual for patients to seek therapy. Some join support groups; others see a therapist privately. In other cases, the caregiver goes to a therapist. Some support groups are open to both caregivers and patients. Others are specifically for family members and caregivers. Ted knew he needed guidance. A few joint sessions with Lois's therapist proved helpful, as were conversations with other caregivers.

Patients want to be whole. They want to return to health, for themselves and for their family and friends. However, because physical and emotional reserves are still low, this internal pressure can slow healing. Stress, anxiety, and fatigue make it more likely patients will lose their tempers or say things they might regret. What should the caregiver do? When the patient takes out her anxiety on the caregiver, should he simply accept the verbal assaults? Does he have the right to express his opinion? If the caregiver does give an opinion, will the partner accuse him of being hypercritical? Doesn't the caregiver have the right and responsibility to respond? If he does respond, is he being unfair? If he doesn't respond, is he treating the patient as someone incapable of communicating? Difficult questions, no simple answers. Ted describes his plight this way: "I don't think about how 'hard' this is on me. I 'just do it.' What are the choices?— walk out of the room when she's venting?—leave dirty dishes in the sink?—let her go to important doctor appointments alone and not get my questions answered?—bring greasy, smelly food into the house when she's nauseous? My decisions are easy."

What is particularly valuable in Ted's story is how a simple e-mail list became not just a chronicle of a disease but a chronicle of connection, a chronicle of life, a chronicle of love. His words motivated others to action. The list gave him an opportunity to express his own emotions. Ted and

Lois learned they needed the skill of the medical professionals when it came to their relationship. They learned they needed the care of friends and family who could help them mend their hearts. To me, the most profound lesson Ted offers is that he and Lois now know that after cancer there is no "normal" normal: "Normal implies some confidence that the road that we have traveled has taught us what to expect around the next bend. That's hubris. What we actually know about the next bend is quite little."

For all of us, we must go forward with the understanding that the next "bend" is unknown. We need to use our energy to explore that path, not to worry about what it may be like. Ted and Lois's experiences remind us of the importance of concrete plans to look forward to—a trip, for example. Plans help the patient to focus on a better future, and sustain hope that normal happy events will continue to be a part of life. If we focus on where we're going in terms of cancer, rather than on where we've been, we can create new paths as Ted and Lois have done.

Cancer changed Lois and Ted. Ted's role was thrust upon him. Near the end of the year, a family member, new to the caregiver role, asked Ted for advice. In capital letters, Ted wrote, "YOU ARE IN CHARGE. Everyone else involved is working for you." Caregivers *are* in charge of those who want to help. We *do* work for them.

It behooves us, therefore, to be as caring and supportive of the caregiver as we are of the patient. If we fail the caregiver, we also fail the patient.

12 REPRISE

"**I** don't know what to say: I don't know what to do." By now we should say those words less frequently. We've seen that there are words and deeds that work, as well as those that fail. The aim is not for perfect behavior, but for better behavior. Most of us will err at some point. However, with practice, we're more likely to know what to say and what to do.

In sports, athletes learn from their mistakes. They need to see their errors if they are to correct them. That's one reason games and practices are videotaped. Players watch themselves and their competitors over and over again. Those positive and negative images become part of their sports persona. Cancer etiquette is not a competition, and our success will be difficult if not impossible to measure. However, just as practice and positive reinforcement lead to success in sports, they also can lead to success when it comes to our giving support at the right time to the people who need it the most.

ETIQUETTE STRATEGIES

- *Stay connected. Stay connected. Stay connected.* If you're not there, you can't help. It's as simple as that.
- Ask. Don't tell.
- If you're not sure what to say, don't say it. Most of our verbal errors are not deliberate.
- If you're not sure what to do, don't do it.
- Wait. If what you say or do will help, it will help a moment or two later.
- It's OK to say you don't know what to say.

- Do your best, but do something. Keep trying.
- If you make a mistake, apologize.
- Take your cues from the patient.
- Listen with eye contact and your full attention.
- Do what you can to help the cancer patient restore some sense of control in his life.
- There are times when silence is the best form of communication.
- Gifts, however small, mean a lot.
- Hugs are good.
- Tell the people you love that you love them. Tell them again and again.
- Remember the caregiver.
- Imagine trading places with the patient. What would you want from family, friends, or colleagues?

This book, *Cancer Etiquette*, is about the impact of cancer on the lives of people we know or love. Cancer causes pain and debilitation, and forces us to acknowledge our mortality. That knowledge, instead of choking us, can help us to celebrate life more. That's the best way to beat cancer: Acknowledge it and stare it down. The patient cannot do it alone. No one can. That's why what we say and what we do can provide life support, in the best sense of the word. What we say and what we do counts for everything.

AFTERWORD
MY PERSONAL CANCER STORY

In 1993, I went in for a routine physical. During the weeks that followed, my internist ordered more tests, including one I had never heard of. Why this particular test? I was a librarian; it was natural for me to research the medical books. The test was one used to diagnose multiple myeloma, cancer of the bone marrow. I read that multiple myeloma was incurable; prognosis, 18 to 24 months. My concern turned to panic. I had never even heard of this disease.

I went to see Dr. Mark Fialk, a hematologist/oncologist, who explained this rare malignancy. Then he said, "Don't laugh when I tell you where you should be treated—Little Rock, Arkansas." I laughed. Less than an hour from the medical Mecca of Manhattan, he told me to travel 1,500 miles for medical care.

Next, I had to tell my children of the diagnosis. It was two hours before I could reach them. Too upset to cry, I vacuumed, washed the floors, did the laundry, and cleaned the kitchen. My cancer clock had started. The next day, a doctor friend spoke with a colleague, and they agreed that the Arkansas Cancer Research Center was the right place for treatment.

My daughter, Leslie, and I flew to Little Rock. After tests, including MRIs, lung and heart evaluations, and the drawing of eleven vials of blood, there was enough information for me to meet with Dr. Bart Barlogie. He discussed options, and gave us unlimited time to ask questions.

With a Stage I diagnosis, I had the option to delay treatment. I chose to start immediately. The first procedure was the insertion of a central line, a Hickman catheter, in my chest. This device—called a port—would be for chemotherapy and the many blood tests that were now in my future. I had a local anesthetic. During the surgery, I talked with the staff about everything from music to fishing. Afterward, the team gave me a small package. In it, I found the retractors and clamps they had used. They said these would be the least painful tools to remove the hook from the fish, an ironic but wonderful way to start the healing process. This small act reminded me that I was not a tumor to them, but a person.

I would have two stem cell transplants, the first as an outpatient. The center required that someone be with me at all times. My daughter, Jean, and my friend, Marilyn, planned itineraries, including Saturday nights for cheaper fares. I couldn't believe that friends and family would be willing to give up vacation time for me. I would be heavily medicated, loaded with hydration bags, weakened, often nauseated, and certainly not good company in any sense of the word.

I plunged into a cancer nether world. There were medical labyrinths to wander through, corridors leading to rooms filled with machines that beeped, hummed, or banged. I learned the language of my cancer. I couldn't even pronounce some of the terms. A humbling moment occurred when the staff gave me a 54-page protocol to sign. On every page, the drugs and their possible side effects were spelled out. This was cancer reality. I had to sign my life away in order to get it back. There was now a cancer calendar as well as a cancer clock.

My daughter, Leslie, was with me one weekend in Little Rock. My hair was falling out in clumps. Only those who have lost their hair, seeing it on their pillows or going down the shower drain, can appreciate the trauma it represents. Some of you may fret over the few hairs coming out on your hairbrush; multiply that a thousand-fold. Imagine what it's like to lose every single hair on your body. In many cases, the eyebrows go, as well as the pubic hair. Hair takes months to grow back, so the cancer patient literally faces the proof of his or her cancer on a daily basis—not for an afternoon, but for what seems like an eternity.

We tried to get a hairdresser to come to the hospital, but could find no one. So Leslie had to cut her mother's hair, and to cut it as close to the scalp as possible. I felt horrible at her having to see me ill, at her having to perform that task. Yet her being there was enormously important to both of us. That particular day is a memory, a gift we still share.

I learned how to do things I never dreamed I was capable of. Cleaning and flushing a catheter was a daily process. Connecting antibiotic vials, never easy, was something I had to do too often. The number of pills I took was enormous. I experienced what people do in their desire to live.

For a year and a half, I had the port in my chest. When I wanted to shower, I had to cover the entire area with plastic, and then tape the plastic securely so no moisture could hit the triple lumen. It took me as long to prepare for the shower as it did to take it. The joy of my first shower without the port was truly immeasurable.

For another four and a half years, I injected myself with a drug, Interferon, three times weekly, something I certainly never expected I'd have to learn to do. I used to say, "Shit!" each time I injected myself. A friend, a touch therapist and someone very much into the power of imaging and meditation, suggested I come up with a better term. I did. I began to say, "L'chaim"—the Hebrew phrase, "To life." You know, it did make a difference.

My religious community was there for me throughout my years of treatment. I still have the hundreds of cards and notes I received; I can't throw them away. One of my favorite memories about the power of community occurred when someone who cared for me took a plane trip. I was in Little Rock, undergoing my first transplant. That particular evening I was alone and feeling very ill. My rabbi and her family were flying to California when the pilot announced that the plane was over Little Rock. Shira immediately called me. That special call, seemingly from the heavens above, served to show me I was being watched over during this terrible period in my life. Finally, after my transplants and the end of chemotherapy, I recovered with a partial remission.

I decided to celebrate with a *bat mitzvah*. This celebration is for girls; *bar mitzvah* is for boys. It is the ritual that welcomes Jewish 13-year olds to life as an adult in the religious community. Girls were not permitted to be *bat mitzvahed* when I was 13, so I decided to do it at age 60. I invited my entire community. My synagogue gave me the gift of a tallis, the traditional prayer shawl. What made this tallis special was that a tape had been sewn into the inner edges, and on that tape many of the congregants had signed their names. Now, whenever I wear the tallis, I am literally wrapped with the good wishes of that community. The day of the *bat mitzvah*, I had only about an inch of hair, yet I refused to wear my wig. I had returned to life; I wasn't going to "cover up" my experience. It was a great day!

I worked until my retirement in 1996. April 2000, I went for a routine mammography. My gynecologist called and asked me to come in for additional pictures. I knew I was in serious trouble when the technician said she would walk those pictures to the radiologist, and my heart sank when my gynecologist came directly into the mammography room. The diagnosis: cancer in both breasts. Nothing had been indicated on my physical examination. Ten years of previous mammographies had been negative.

Double biopsies confirmed the diagnosis. Thanks to the marvels of medical science, I had survived long enough to develop a second cancer. There were now two cancer clocks running. My personal double whammy.

Because of my history, the treatment decision was complicated. Dr. Sundar Jagannath, one of my doctors in Little Rock, had moved to New York City to head the transplant unit at the St. Vincent's Comprehensive Cancer Center. I went to see him. Dr. Jagannath walked with me to meet the radiologist whose specialty was breast cancer. Later, I consulted with Dr. Paula Klein, a breast oncologist. These physicians were doing everything possible to help me through this latest crisis. Dr. Fialk, who is still my oncologist, joined in the consultations.

The period from mammography to surgery was about five weeks. The day my daughter, Jean, gave birth to her son, I had to tell her of the biopsy results and the need for a double mastectomy. I then told Leslie, who was also pregnant. Those were calls I never dreamed I would have to make again.

Dr. Mark Gordon, my surgeon, was attentive and concerned. He treated me as someone who had to deal with a second primary cancer, as well as a double mastectomy. I had to ask for help again. My community rallied once more.

We set the date for surgery. When I awoke from the anesthesia, my daughter Jean was there stroking my forehead and saying, "I love you, Mom." Only two weeks before, she had given birth to her son, Henry. She was able to be with me because my daughter Leslie's in-laws waited with Jean during the long hours of surgery. They stayed with the baby when Jean was finally allowed to see me, late that evening. Jean did not have to be alone, and I did not have to be alone. Only later did I learn how many hours the in-laws, Fran and George, were there.

My surgery was in late May. A few months later, I started chemotherapy, four rounds of Taxol, which lasted six months. The treatment, although unpleasant, was relatively uneventful. What was most memorable, however, was the last day of treatment.

As usual, I walked to the hospital. That 15-minute walk was not just a bit of exercise; it was my way of asserting control. I hadn't asked anyone for a ride. I was on my own. At White Plains Hospital, 5F is the cancer treatment floor. An outpatient room can accommodate four patients, but on this particular hot September day, I was alone. Michelle would be in charge of my treatment, and she greeted me with her usual smile and hug.

Years ago, I hadn't worried when the technicians had to find a vein. Then, my veins were strong, and the needle stick was usually easy. However, the breast cancer chemotherapy presented a particular problem. In early June, only days after my breast surgery, I tried to open a window in my apartment. I accidentally banged my left arm and developed a huge black and blue mark, a hematoma. That caused lymphedema, or swelling, in the arm. This was particularly upsetting because I was left-handed. Lymphedema can be serious and permanent. I had to undergo weeks of physical therapy to lessen its effects.

Breast cancer literature says that a patient who has had a mastectomy should have blood work drawn and blood pressure taken from the other arm. What should a patient who has a double mastectomy do? It was a crapshoot. I worried each time I had to have a needle inserted. I worried about the technician's ability to find a good vein in my arm. Would the stick cause another lymphedema problem? With every treatment, I worried. The technician needed two attempts, but the IV was started. Michelle stayed with me during what ordinarily would be a very simple procedure. She knew her presence reduced my anxiety. The needle went in; the stick was over.

This morning seemed no different from any of the other treatment days. My usual routine, once the IV started, was to read *The New York Times*. Then I'd attempt the crossword puzzle. Later my choice would be a mystery tape or book. I would be in the chair for about five hours. At times, I'd wend my way, clutching the IV pole, to go to the bathroom. With luck, I might be able to doze a bit, usually a side effect from one or more of the drugs. There would then be a nondescript lunch, various checks on vital signs, and occasional problems with the flow of the drugs, which included Taxol, steroids, anti-nausea drugs, and Benadryl. The setting was the same; there were the recliners, the chairs, the television, and the oxygen lines. The beep of the computerized IV would be a constant.

This last chemo was a transforming experience. Yes, it was still a hospital room, but it felt like home. My first visitor was Lennie, a friend and hospital volunteer. He dropped in to tell me about how his morning was going. After he left, Michelle, still monitoring my vital signs and medications, needed to talk. We spoke then as friends, not patient and nurse. Michelle, who had been one of my oncology nurses since my diagnosis for multiple myeloma, needed some TLC from *me*. I didn't know the right words for what she was facing, and admitted it. But the words weren't important. What she needed, and what I could give, were a welcome ear and a caring heart. I could listen. I gave her my full attention. Even in the hospital room, she saw me not as a cancer, but as a person with whom she could talk.

The hours passed. Trish, who took over when Michelle's shift ended, came in. Trish was always upbeat, always joyful. She told me she had completed the questionnaire I had given her for this book. Then she turned serious. She told me about one of her patients, a 29-year old breast cancer patient who was critically ill. Obviously, she didn't mention the patient's name. To complicate matters, Trish's best friend, only 32 years old, recently had a double mastectomy. This nurse who devotes her life to those with cancer was struggling with her emotions. "I don't know what to do," she said. Sometimes words fail even the best of us.

Yet, in this transformed space, for a few moments at least, she could tell me of her pain and frustration, her inability to deal with the reality of cancer. I could listen; I was there for her, as she had been there so many, many times for me. Although Trish may have thought her words failed, her presence with the patient never did.

We spoke. Would simply holding her patient's hand help? Part of the problem was that the young woman did not know the full extent of her illness. It really wasn't any specific advice Trish wanted from me. She needed to talk of her pain as both a professional caregiver and friend. She knew she could acknowledge her emotional overload to me. Trish's identification with her dear friend who was so young and who had breast cancer, and her concern for the young patient on floor 5F intensified her stress. My room now was more than a treatment room; it had become a place of connection, of sharing, of giving, of communication. The drip of the IV was the medical healing. Our words were the symbolic healing. What I said was unimportant. I focused on Trish. I was there for her.

A few minutes later, Christina, the hospital chaplain, stopped in on her tour of the floor. We had been on a panel together for the Leukemia & Lymphoma Society, and had gotten to know each other then. Christina knew I was working on a book about cancer. We spoke about a presentation on survivorship she was to do that evening. Trish again came in to check and see how I was feeling. The three of us spoke of the difficulty of communicating about cancer. It's as though I were in my kitchen at home, and friends were dropping in for a chat.

Eloise, a good friend who was to take me home after my treatment, arrived at about 2 p.m. Eloise is an artist. She said she wanted to sharpen her skills with charcoal, especially portraits. I was wearing my baseball cap, having decided against wearing my wig that very warm day. She began to sketch. The sketch captured me, bald and wan though I was. This was amazing to me because my self-image had never been a very positive one. Yet within minutes, Eloise had drawn an image of me that I could accept. My spirit was in that charcoal. It was a great gift.

The IV finished; the computer stopped its rhythmic beeps. When Trish removed the IV and cleaned the injection site, I was finished with what I hoped was the last cancer treatment I would ever have. I went into the bathroom. Within seconds, I heard voices, and a knock on the bathroom door. "I'll be right out," I said. When I opened the door, there in the room, applauding my end of treatment, were all the oncology nurses from 5F. They gave me a gift, a small framed picture of a wooded scene. Underneath the image were the words, "Yesterday is but a dream. Tomorrow, a vision of hope. Look to this day for it is life." There they all were, celebrating *my* life.

So that day, that last chemo day, in a room where drugs were destroying the cells in my body, I was recalled to life. Everyone who had stepped into that room on that day had seen me as whole, not broken. Everyone who had been with me that day was part of my community. As with life, during those hours, even though there was pain and frustration, there was connection and love.

In recalling that day, I remember a powerful story that Eda LeShan, a psychologist, wrote in *Woman's Day* about her 59th birthday. LeShan tells of the friend who asked her if she knew how lobsters grow. The friend said that a lobster grows only if it sheds its shell regularly. He must find a safe area to shed his shell, and at this stage is in danger and vulnerable to attack. LeShan writes, "In other words, a lobster has to risk its life in order to grow."

The lobster can be a metaphor for those of us who have cancer. As patients, we have to shed our cancer shell. Treatment makes us vulnerable to infection. We shed our hair and our body changes, often permanently. However if we don't shed our cancer shell, if we don't grow new life shells, we will die. I had to shed several shells in order to survive, but I have, and I have grown—though not without a struggle.

Cancer is more than a medical fender bender. Its impact is forever. In my case, I've had 20 bone marrow biopsies, surgical insertion and removal of three ports used for treatment, stem cell transplants, and high-dose chemotherapy that lasted for months and months. High-dose chemotherapy, before transplant, is meant to kill as many cancer cells as possible. Those drugs are not yet capable of sidestepping the good cells, so the digestive system, the immune system, and virtually every muscle and bone in the body are affected. The pain was severe at times.

Because the white blood count must be brought down to zero, death from infection is a real possibility. I once used an emery board during the transplant process. An infection developed, and I needed minor surgery on the affected finger. Mouth sores and thrush can be excruciating. I lost my hair not once but three times. My experiences are not unique.

Christina Middlebrook in *Seeing the Crab* writes of cancer as a battle. She speaks of bombardment, an interesting term if one thinks of radiation and chemotherapy. To her, cancer is trench warfare. In a brilliant image of a hostage situation, she describes how difficult it is to deal with cancer. The captors take the hostage to the courtyard and blindfold him. The hostage sees the firing squad and expects to be shot. Instead of hearing the crack of the bullet, the hostage is returned to his cell. This trauma may be repeated again and again as a form of torture. As a patient, I face the cancer firing squad before every biopsy, MRI, or blood test. Will this test mean execution? Even if the execution is stayed, I will face the firing squad with every major checkup.

Am I the same person I was before I dealt with cancer? I don't think so. Was I a terrible person before? No. It's that my "To Do" list, my map, has changed. Cancer sends shock waves through us. If we see cancer only as a trauma and not a wakeup call, we've missed a major opportunity in our life. The wakeup call need not mean dramatic life changes. It may be a decision to spend more time with friends and family. It may mean more time to play, or—as the cliché goes—"smell the roses." It may mean a return to a lifelong love of painting. It may mean reconnection to church or synagogue. It may mean becoming pro-active for a cause you always believed in. It has to mean something. As Arthur Frank writes, ". . . recovery is worth only as much as what you learn about the life you are regaining."

Cancer transforms. Obviously, it has a physical impact. Its effect on the soul is no less profound. No one remains the same—not the patient, caregivers, family, friends, or coworkers. I went home after that last treatment knowing that connection can occur in the most unexpected places and in the most unexpected ways. Everyone's efforts are needed for true healing to occur. The medical staff's responsibility is the physical. We expect proactive doctors, nurses, and technicians. Their tools are scalpel and drugs. Our tools are words and deeds—different—but no less potent.

WITH APPRECIATION

I have so much to be thankful for. Sometimes I don't think we thank people enough for what they have given us. At least, I can acknowledge those who have played a role in my journey with this book.

I will be forever grateful to Harriet Ross, my editor, for believing in and understanding what this book was aiming to do; and with her high standards, directing her editorial skills to shape my manuscript into the kind of book I hoped it could be.

I am indebted to my medical community. Dr. Marvin Lipman, a skilled diagnostician, caught the multiple myeloma in its earliest stage and referred me to an oncologist, Dr. Mark Fialk. He is still the physician to whom I turn first, and whose medical judgment I totally trust.

The Arkansas Cancer Research Center is an extraordinary place. Once I consulted with Dr. Bart Barlogie, I knew that was where I wanted to receive treatment. To everyone there, I thank you for your talent and for your caring.

After Dr. Sundar Jagannath, who treated me in Little Rock, became Chief of the Multiple Myeloma and Blood and Bone Marrow Transplantation Program at the St. Vincent's Comprehensive Cancer Center in New York, I went to him for my myeloma checkups. When I was diagnosed with breast cancer, this extraordinary doctor guided me to Dr. Paula Klein the breast cancer oncologist at St. Vincent's. Thanks also to Stephanie Stoss, Multiple Myeloma-Transplant Program Manager.

For more then ten years, I have received excellent care at the White Plains Hospital Medical Center. Dr. Mark Gordon, my surgeon, has compassion as well as talent. I thank everyone associated with the hospital, especially those who work on 5F. Kathy Duffy, Administrative Director, Cancer Program, has always been there for me when I needed advice. Joan Milano has guided me through many issues.

I have been blessed with many friends and family members who were with me throughout my cancer struggles. I won't name them all, but I want to recognize my Little Rock Alumni who came to stay with me during my treatment there. I could not have done it without you—Janel

Halpern, Rita Barasch, Marilyn Menack, Judy Wiener, Ginette Wachtel, David Molot, Joan Ostacher, Carol Caro, Gloria Horowitz, and my sister, Harriet Brown.

Susan Gordon became my mentor. She taught me that writing and rewriting are part of the trade, and that frustration is a normal part of the writer's life. Rita Silverman, Lorna Greenberg, and others made valuable suggestions to me as I worked on the manuscript. All tried to help me get through the anxieties about my writing.

Thanks to the librarians and staff at Westchester Community College in Valhalla, New York. They were always available when I needed an interlibrary loan, or if I needed an article available only on microfilm.

Thank you, Judith Rivin. Thanks to the Milgrom-Elcott family for making me a part of their lives. To Shira Milgrom, my Rabbi and friend, you have been a blessing. I thank Rabbi Edie Mencher whose ability to make me laugh and think is amazing.

A special note of thanks to Linda and Joel Negrin for their generosity in baring their private lives so that others in their situation might benefit from their experiences. I cannot ever thank enough those who shared their stories with me. I feel as though I know many of you. You sent me your stories of love and of pain, of joy and of disappointment. Every one of your experiences taught me about how cancer, "the crab," crawls into every aspect of our lives, and how even though we may not be cured, we can heal.

I need to say that without my daughters, Jean and Leslie, and Rick Molot and Alan Wolfe, the loves of their lives, I may not have had the will or the strength to go on. David, I think of you every day.

Alex, Sidney, Josh, Maddie, and Henry will probably not read the book at this point in their lives. Being their grandmother has been extraordinary for me. Hugging and loving them has been the best medicine.

I thank you all.

—R.K.

RESOURCES

Albert, Louise. *Less Than Perfect*, New York: Holiday House, 2003.

Altman, Lawrence K. "Study Suggests Overuse of Chemotherapy Near Life's End." *The New York Times* 13 May 2001, late ed.: A 22.

Ames, Lynne. "Swimming and Raising Money for Pediatric Cancer." *The New York Times* 25 Aug. 2002, late ed.: WE 7.

Anderson, Dave. "The Babe Returned From Cancer." *The New York Times* 20 May 2004, late ed.: D7.

Armstrong, Lance. *It's Not About the Bike: My Journey Back to Life*. Thorndike, ME: Thorndike Press, 2000.

Babcock, Elise NeeDell. *When Life Becomes Precious: A Guide for Loved Ones and Cancer Patients.* New York: Bantam Books, 1997.

Biro, David. *One Hundred Days.* New York: Pantheon Books, 2000.

Bloch, Annette and Richard. *Fighting Cancer.* Kansas City, MO: R.A. Bloch Cancer Foundation, 1990.

Bombeck, Erma. *I Want to Grow Hair, I Want to Grow Up, I Want to Go to Boise.* New York: Harper and Row, 1989.

Brody, Jane E. "Art and Grace, When It's Time to Say Goodbye." *The New York Times* 30 Dec. 2003, late ed.: F6.

———. "A Doctor's Story of Hope, Humor and Deadly Cancer." *The New York Times* 15 May 2001, late ed.: F5+.

———. "For Patients in the Hospital, the Good Visitor Can Play an Important Role in Recovery." *The New York Times* 14 May 1986, late ed.: C10.

Buckman, Robert. *I Don't Know What to Say: How to Help and Support Someone Who is Dying.* Toronto: Key Porter Books, 1988.

Burton, Susan. "About a Doll." *The New York Times Magazine* 29 Dec. 2002, 11.

Christakis, Nicholas. "A Doctor With a Cause: 'What's my Prognosis?' " *The New York Times* 28 Nov. 2000, late ed.: F7.

Clifford, Christine. *Cancer Has Its Privileges: Stories of Hope and Laughter.* New York: Berkley Publishing, 2002.

Cohen, Deborah and Robert M. Gelfand. *Just Get Me Through This.* New York: Kensington Books, 2000.

Cole, Diane. "Words That Help, Words That Hurt." *Intouch* July 2001: 41–44.

Cooke, Margaret. *Ways You Can Help.* New York: Warner Books, 1996.

Cousins, Norman. *Anatomy of an Illness.* New York: Norton, 1979.

Davis, Amelia. *The First Look.* Chicago: University of Illinois Press, 2000.

Dreifus, Claudia. "Promising Judgments That Are Purely Medical." *The New York Times* 18 June 2002, late ed.: F6.

Dunne, Dominick. "Another Party, Another Clue." *Vanity Fair*. March 2001: 148–157.

Edson, Margaret. *Wit*. New York: Faber and Faber, Inc., 1999.

Fine, Saralee and Robert Fine. *Prostate Cancer: A Doctor's Personal Triumph*. Forest Dale, VT: Paul S. Eriksson, 1999.

Finn, Robin. "Doctor For Giuliani Has an Artist's Touch." *The New York Times* 22 Sept. 2000, late ed.: B2.

Frank, Arthur. *At the Will of the Body*. Boston: Houghton Mifflin Company, 1991.

Greaves, Mel. *Cancer: The Evolutionary Legacy*. London: Oxford University Press, 2000.

Gamarekian, Barbara. "Finding Moments of Comfort and Humor While Facing Cancer Treatment." *The New York Times* 27 Aug. 2002, late ed.: F7.

Groopman, Jerome. *The Anatomy of Hope*. New York: Random House, 2004.

———. *The Measure of Our Days*. New York: Viking, 1997.

Guilmartin, Nance. *Healing Conversations*. San Francisco: Jossey-Bass, 2002.

Hammerschmidt, Rosalie and Clifton K. Meador. *A Little Book of Nurses' Rules*. Philadelphia: Hanley and Belfus, Inc., 1993.

Handler, Evan. *Time on Fire*. New York: Little Brown and Co., 1996.

Harwell, Amy. *When Your Friend Gets Cancer*. Wheaton, IL: Harold Shaw Publishers, 1987.

Hoffman, Alice. "Sustained By Fiction While Facing Life's Facts." *The New York Times* 14 Aug. 2000, late ed.: E1–2.

Holland, Jimmie. *The Human Side of Cancer*. New York: Harper Collins, 2001.

Hollenberg, Emily. "Top 11 Ways to Know You Are a Cancer Survivor." Comprehensive Cancer Center, University of Michigan. <8 Sept. 2004; http://p53.cancer.med.umich.edu/share/humorten.htm>

Honeyman, Catharine. "Humor." Comprehensive Cancer Center, University of Michigan Humor. <8 Sept. 2004; www.cancer.med.umich.edu/share/brighthum.htm.>

Ivins, Molly. "Who Needs Breasts, Anyway?" *Time*. 18 Feb. 2002: 58.

Jenkins, Lee. "Baylor Is Back at Camp After Cancer Treatment." *The New York Times* 22 March 2004, late ed.: D8.

Jordan, Hanilton. *No Such Thing As a Bad Day*. Marietta, GA: Longstreet Press, 2000.

Keary, Lila. "When Good Intentions Happen to Bad Problems." *Oprah* Feb. 2001: 108+.

King, Dean, Jessica King, and Jonathon Pearlroth. *Cancer Combat*. New York: Bantam Books, 1998.

Klein, Allen. *The Courage to Laugh*. New York: Penguin Putnam, Inc., 1998.

Kolata, Gina. "A Doctor With a Cause: What's My Prognosis?" *The New York Times* 28 Nov. 2000, late ed.: F7.

———. "In One Word, an Entire Debate on Cancer." *The New York Times* 1 June 2004, late ed.: A14.

———. "New Approach About Cancer and Survival." *The New York Times* 1 June 2004, late ed.: A1+

Korda, Michael. *Man to Man: Surviving Prostate Cancer*. Thorndike, ME: Thorndike Press, 1996.

Kushner, Laurence. *Honey from the Rock*. Woodstock, Vt.: Jewish Lights, 1992.

Landro, Laura. Survivor: *Taking Control of Your Fight Against Cancer*. New York: Simon and Schuster, 1998.

LaTour, Kathy. "Cancer Survivorship." *Cure*. Summer 2003: 6.

Langone, John. "Medical Schools Discover Value in Dispensing Compassion." *The New York Times* 22 Aug. 2000, late ed.: F7.

Lemonick, Michael D. and Alice Park. "New Hope for Cancer." *Time* 28 May 2001: 62–69.

Leopold, Ellen. *A Darker Ribbon. Breast Cancer: Women and Their Doctors in the Twentieth Century.* Boston: Beacon Press, 1999.

Lerner, Barron. "In the Death of a Doctor, a Lesson" *The New York Times* 23 July 2002, late ed.: F4.

LeShan, Eda. "The Risk of Growing." *Woman's Day* 22 Sept. 1981: 26.

Lipsyte, Robert. *In the Country of Illness: Comfort and Advice for the Journey.* New York: Knopf, 1998.

Lombardi, Kate Stone. "Chaplains as Comforters and Counselors." *The New York Times* 20 July 2003, late ed.: WE 1.

Marcus, Amy Dockser. "Cancer Fights Shifts to Survivors." *The Wall Street Journal* 24 March 2004, D1+.

Marks, Peter. "The Laugh Lab at Carnegie Hall." *The New York Times* 10 Oct. 2001, late ed.: E1.

McKenna, Julie. "Richard Crenna." *Coping* May/June 2001:8–9.

Middlebrook, Christina. *Seeing the Crab: A Memoir of Dying.* New York: Basic Books, 1996.

Murphy, Beth. *Fighting For Our Future. How Young Women Find Strength, Hope, and Courage While Taking Control of Breast Cancer.* New York: McGraw-Hill 2003.

Nash, Jennie. *Victoria's Secret Catalog Never Stops Coming: And Other Lessons I Learned from Breast Cancer.* New York: Simon & Schuster, 2001.

Nathan, Joel. *What To Do When They Say "It's Cancer".* St. Leonards, Australia: Allen & Unwin, 1999.

Ness, Erik. "The Mummy's Tumor." *MAMM* October 2000:49–51.

Nielsen, Jerri. *Ice Bound.* New York: Hyperion, 2001.

NIH US Department of Health and Human Services, National Institutes of Health. *Taking Time.* Bethesda, MD: National Cancer Institute, 1986.

O'Donnell, Rosie and Deborah Axelrod. *Bosom Buddies.* New York: Warner Books, 1999.

Ogle, Kathleen M. "Sometimes, the Doctor is Blind." *The New York Times* 6 Nov. 2001, late ed.: F5.

Perez-Peña, Richard. "Hair Styling, Plus Cancer Education." *The New York Times* 6 Nov. 2003, late ed.: B1

Peaboody, Francis Weld. *The Care of the Patient.* Boston: Harvard University Press, 1956.

Picardie, Ruth. *Before I Say Goodbye.* New York: Henry Holt & Co., 2000.

Porter, Margit Esser. *The Breast Cancer Treatment Survival Handbook.* New York: Simon and Schuster, 1997.

Porter, Margit Esser. *Hope Lives: The After Breast Cancer Treatment Survival Handbook.* Peterborough, NH: Hic Publishing, 2000.

Radner, Gilda. *It's Always Something.* New York: Simon and Schuster, 1989.

Ratner, Elaine. *The Feisty Woman's Breast Cancer Book.* Alameda, CA.: Hunter House, Inc., 1999.

Redgrave, Lynn. "Our Journal." *The New York Times Magazine*. 18 April 2004., Section 6, 36–41.

Remen, Rachel Naomi. *My Grandfather's Blessings*. New York: Riverhead Books, 2000.

Ritchie, Karen. "Angels and Bolters: A Field Guide to the Wildlife of Cancer." *CancerLynx* 8 May 2000. <8 Sept. 2004; http://www.cancerlynx..com/angels_bolters.html>

Ryan, Dick. *Straight From the Heart*. New York: Crossroad Publishing Company, 2001.

Schimmel, Selma with Barry Fox. *Cancer Talk*. New York: Broadway Books, 1999.

Severo, Richard. "Steve Allen, Comedian Who Pioneered Late-Night TV Talk Shows, is Dead at 78." *The New York Times* 1 Nov. 2000, late ed.: B13.

Severo, Richard. "Harold Russell Dies at 88; Veteran and Oscar Winner." *The New York Times* 1 Feb. 2002, late ed.: B9.

Shapiro, Dan. *Mom's Marijuana*. New York: Harmony Books, 2000.

Shaywitz, David A. "The Right to Live." *The New York Times* 19 Sept. 2000, late ed.: A 25.

Siegel, Bernie S. *How to Live Between Office Visits*. New York: Harper Collins, 1993.

———. *Love, Medicine & Miracles*. New York: Harper & Row, 1990

Sontag, Susan. *Illness As Metaphor*. New York: Farrar, Straus and Giroux, 1977.

Spiegel, David. *Living Beyond Limits*. New York: Times Books, 1993.

Spingarn, Natalie Davis. *The New Cancer Survivors*. Baltimore: Johns Hopkins University Press, 1999.

Spizman, Robyn Freedman. *When Words Matter Most*. New York: Crown Publishers Inc., 1996.

Stephenson, Jane, Katz, Michael S. et al. "Cancer Care: What Are the Priorities?" *The Lancet* October 2001: 636–41.

Stevens, Barbara F. *Not Just One in Eight*. Deerfield Beach, FL: Health Communications, 2000.

Stronach, Karen. *Survivors' Guide for Bone Marrow/Stem Cell Transplant*. Southfield, MI: NBMTLink, 2002.

Telushkin, Joseph. *Words That Hurt, Words That Heal: How to Choose Words Wisely and Well*. New York: William Morrow & Co., 1996.

Tillman, David. *In the Failing Light*. Berkeley, CA.: Creative Arts Book Company, 1999.

Tommasini, Anthony. "A Thank You to Medicine from Spunky Survivors." *The New York Times* 27 Sep. 2000, late ed.: E7.

Trillin, Alice Stewart. "Betting Your Life." *The New Yorker* 29 Jan. 2001: 38–42.

———. "Of Dragons and Garden Peas." *The New England Journal of Medicine* 304 (1981): 699–701.

Ubel, Peter A. "A Fine Line Between Ask and Tell." *The New York Times* 13 April 2004, late ed.: F5.

Villarosa, Linda. "Doctors With Sick Parents See a System's Flaws." *The New York Times* 16 Oct. 2001, late ed.: F5.

Wilber, Ken. *Grace and Grit*. Boston: Shambhala, 1993.

Woo, Elaine. "Ruth Handler, Inventor of Barbie Doll, Dies at 85." *Los Angeles Times* latimes.com. 28 April 2002. < 8 Sept. 2004; http://www.latimes.com/la-042802handler.story.>

Wyatt, Richard J. "Words to Live By." *Washington Post*. 13 Feb. 2001, HE16 <8 March 2001; http://washingtonpost.com/wp-dyn/health/A51505-2001Feb9.html>